Transforming Health Care Management

Integrating Technology Strategies

Ivan J. Barrick, PhD, FACHE, CPHIMS

Assistant Professor
Adjunct Faculty
University of Southern Indiana
Pennsylvania State University
University of Scranton

JONES AND BARTLETT PUBLISHERS
Sudbury, Massachusetts
BOSTON   TORONTO   LONDON   SINGAPORE

World Headquarters

Jones and Bartlett Publishers	Jones and Bartlett Publishers	Jones and Bartlett Publishers
40 Tall Pine Drive	Canada	International
Sudbury, MA 01776	6339 Ormindale Way	Barb House, Barb Mews
978-443-5000	Mississauga, Ontario L5V 1J2	London W6 7PA
info@jbpub.com	Canada	UK
www.jbpub.com		

Jones and Bartlett's books and products are available through most bookstores and online book-sellers. To contact Jones and Bartlett Publishers directly, call 800-832-0034, fax 978-443-8000, or visit our website www.jbpub.com.

Substantial discounts on bulk quantities of Jones and Bartlett's publications are available to corporations, professional associations, and other qualified organizations. For details and specific discount information, contact the special sales department at Jones and Bartlett via the above contact information or send an email to specialsales@jbpub.com.

This publication is designed to provide accurate and authoritative information in regard to the Subject Matter covered. It is sold with the understanding that the publisher is not engaged in rendering legal, accounting, or other professional service. If legal advice or other expert assistance is required, the service of a competent professional person should be sought.

Production Credits

Publisher: Michael Brown
Production Director: Amy Rose
Associate Editor: Katey Birtcher
Production Editor: Tracey Chapman
Production Assistant: Roya Millard
Marketing Manager: Sophie Fleck
Manufacturing Buyer: Therese Connell

Composition: Publishers' Design and Production Services, Inc.
Cover Design: Kate Ternullo
Cover Image: © Krishnacreations/ShutterStock, Inc.
Printing and Binding: Malloy, Inc.
Cover Printing: Malloy, Inc.

Library of Congress Cataloging-in-Publication Data
Barrick, Ivan.
    Transforming health care management : integrating technology strategies/Ivan Barrick.
        p. ; cm.
    Includes bibliographical references.
    ISBN 978-0-7637-4450-2 (alk. paper)
    1. Health services administration—Data processing.   2. Information resources management.
3. Information storage and retrieval systems—Public health.   I. Title.
    [DNLM: 1. Health Services Administration. 2. Information Management. 3. Management Information Systems.   W 84.1 B275t 2008]
    RA971.23.B37 2008
    362.10285—dc22
                                                                                2007035187
6048

Printed in the United States of America
12 11 10 09 08   10 9 8 7 6 5 4 3 2 1

Dedication

This book is dedicated to my family; without their support throughout my career, this book would not be a reality.

Additionally, I owe considerable gratitude to those dedicated leaders and pioneers throughout the healthcare industry and medical military community who educated, mentored, and counseled me during the last forty years. Their contributions of shared experience, insight, and expertise enabled me to achieve success and rebound from failure during my career.

Contents

About the Author

IVAN BARRICK, PHD, FACHE, CPHIMS

As an assistant professor and an adjunct faculty member at the University of Southern Indiana, Pennsylvania State University, and the University of Scranton, Dr. Barrick taught health services administration, information management, and operations research graduate and undergraduate courses.

As Director of Parente Randolph's Healthcare Operations Improvement Practice, Dr. Barrick was responsible for process reengineering, operations research and his process improvement engagements, productivity management, staffing and related due diligence assessments, quality management audits, benchmarking, organization development, information systems, strategic planning engagements, HIPAA administration simplification compliance assessments, and remediation projects.

Dr. Barrick consulted with and was employed by academic medical enters, community hospitals, integrated healthcare systems, post-acute systems, medical groups, health management organizations, psychiatric hospitals, Veterans Administration, and military facilities.

He has served on boards of directors of regional healthcare, human service organizations, and as vice president of a Regional WEDI-SNIP affiliate, the e-Pennsylvania Alliance. Throughout a thirty-five year career in health care, Dr. Barrick held a number of positions. These positions include president of an independent healthcare operations improvement consultancy, Chief Information Officer, director of corporate, line, and staff functions in large academic medical centers, hospitals, and health systems. Extensive administrative, management consulting, clinical, and technical experience brings unique healthcare delivery perspectives. In addition, he served as CIO for Navy Bureau of Medicine and Surgery in a Combat Zone Fleet Hospital, retiring as a Commander, Medical Service Corps, United States Naval Reserve.

Dr. Barrick earned a Doctorate in Healthcare Administration, a Masters degree in Public Administration, and a Bachelor of Science degree in Medical Technology.

He has published extensively in professional journals, co-authored several books, and contributed to several healthcare textbook chapters.

He is credentialed as a Fellow in the College of Healthcare Executives, a Certified Healthcare Information Management Professional, and the American Society of Clinical Pathology as a medical technologist.

Preface

Health care is a very troubled industry!

Peter Drucker and other operations management experts have characterized healthcare organizations and hospitals as the "most complex, barely manageable places [. . .] maybe the most complex organizations in human history." Health care is not a "seamless system" or even one in which a designer, operator, user, manager, or customer view a process or a system from a common perspective. As an active participant in designing, implementing, managing, changing, and training in healthcare operations and systems for more that three decades, I agree with management experts and conclude that the problems in our healthcare industry are no real surprise. For more than a quarter century, my responsibilities have included those of an educator, a chief information officer (CIO), a management engineer, an operations consultant and analyst, a civilian executive and military officer, a division director and clinician, and, most importantly, a patient.

Recognizing that healthcare organizations are so complex, should we really expect that any process or system in these confounding environments could be perceived any differently? As educators we are challenged to prepare our students, our nation's next generation of healthcare leaders. Today's students will be rapidly tasked to design, implement, manage, operate, monitor, and improve technology, processes, and programs. They will assess systems and process effectiveness using these key tools and techniques typically embedded in programs such as quality leadership, continuous process improvement, process redesign through reengineering, clinical process and system protocol redesign, or, most contemporarily, Six Sigma, lean enterprise, and organizational transformation. We cannot fulfill our educational obligation unless our aspiring professionals speak the same language.

Those of us directly involved in this industry-wide digital transformation process must encourage the use of standardized knowledge with a common vocabulary that incorporates essential elements of all technology-driven clinical disciplines. As an industry we have just begun to understand that digitized medical records can only be effectively used when built and maintained with a nationally standardized infrastructure.

Until now, a fundamental problem for both educators and students was that this book had yet to be written. Recognizing this unmet need, this primer is offered as fundamental tool for key healthcare process, systems, or technology stakeholders. This textbook takes initial steps in this clearly focused direction.

As both clinicians and administrators, we practice in an industry that represents more than 20% of America's economy. We are all simultaneously challenged to deliver safe, cost-effective, consumer-friendly care and to do so while being digitally transformed. As educators, as students, and as those producing educational materials we must promote a multidisciplinary understanding of essential concepts relevant to all information technology (IT) disciplines, such as management engineering, systems analysis, networks, communications, and information systems.

Although frequently critical of "bureaucratic hospital silos" of the independent nursing, laboratory, pharmacy, and other departments, we naively fail to acknowledge or clearly understand that we have our own "silos" embedded within and among our IT disciplines.

Technology and process transformational concepts are presented in a language so that students at all levels can understand, articulate, and demonstrate fundamental competence, knowledge, language, and vocabulary in these essential subject areas:

- Information Systems
- Information Systems Design
- Information Systems Analysis
- Management Engineering
- Operations Research
- Operations Analysis
- Clinical Informatics
- Networking and Communications
- Business Process Engineering
- Six Sigma
- Lean Enterprise
- Quality Management
- Quality Leadership
- Project Management and Work Breakdown Structure
- Productivity Management and Performance Improvement

Anyone planning a career in these areas can relate to health care's administrative and clinical processes and can understand them from a patient's perspective, having experienced these error-prone processes in healthcare encounters. As each student explores these processes, systems, and IT concepts from this integrated perspective, value analysis is enhanced when viewed from circumstances that have impacted his or her own life. This approach offers increased potential for more understanding and greater retention of key concepts.

This textbook is designed for study in management engineering, computer systems, and healthcare IT programs and maintains an increased level of rigor common in Association of University Programs in Hospital Administration (AUPHA) accredited undergraduate programs and Commission on Accreditation of Healthcare Management Education (CAHME) accredited graduate programs. Operations research and IT topics are, by definition, technical subjects, and they are presented to complement each individual discipline's curriculum goals.

The language, tone, and graphics are presented like those of an introductory textbook, but they are rigorous enough to meet stringent academic accreditation standards. The key concepts and applications presented here both prepare students to credibly discuss healthcare systems and to enlighten process and IT professionals desiring to learn more technical aspects of these subjects. Our subject matter is laden with fundamentally essential clinical, engineering, and systems technical terms that can be quite intimidating when first encountered, but throughout this text we introduce and explain these terms.

This book is a primer for healthcare IT, operations research, systems analysis, process improvement, and informatics students. Additionally, this text will interest instructors teaching discipline-specific audiences in clinical specialty undergraduate programs (e.g., digital imaging nursing, medical technology, etc.). Medical students intending to pursue a career in the rapidly evolving field of medical informatics may be interested as well.

Chapters are structured and sequenced within five major sections. The first section introduces a focused rationale and common approach within four chapters:

- Digitally Transforming Health Care: An Introduction
- Multidisciplinary Concepts: A Fundamental Foundation
- Information Technology: Components, Functions, and Features
- Networking to Digitally Transform Healthcare Communications

The second section builds on this foundation and expands content scope and topic depth initially introduced, while preparing for more advanced topics:

- Quality Management
- Process Redesign Strategies
- Transformational Strategies for Tactical Project Management

The third section further develops these topics from a more comprehensive multidisciplinary approach to traditional operations research, process and performance improvement concepts, and quantitative analytical tools and techniques:

- Tactical Work Breakdown and Workload Analysis
- Productivity Measurement and Performance Management
- Queuing Theory and Waiting Line Analysis

Techniques used to achieve effective digital transformation of critical care delivery processes are highlighted in the fourth section:

- Process Simulation and Predictive Modeling
- Strategic Application of Six Sigma Concepts
- Tactical Application of Lean Enterprise Theory

The last section incorporates the fundamental techniques presented earlier and more advanced concepts and essential strategies to lead digital transformation initiatives. This section highlights pioneering experiences and futurists' expectations for patient-centric healthcare delivery capabilities and challenges of foreseeable applications:

- Telemedicine and Clinical Informatics
- Emerging Technologies
- Visionary Perspectives: Healthcare's Future, 2014 and Beyond

With a primary focus on a relatively junior audience, this text encourages students to develop an accelerating recognition of IT, process reengineering, and digital redesign strategies to drive the digital transformation of the industry in virtually every healthcare profession's programs. It is an excellent supplement to existing management-related course texts in clinical programs to incorporate process analysis, quality management (QM), process improvement, and Six Sigma and Lean Enterprise concepts in healthcare organizations that are expanding continuing education programs. Content specifically addresses fundamental, discipline-specific, and integrated subject areas essential to aspiring professionals faced with a rapidly accelerating demand for digitized healthcare organizations of all types and venues.

Of necessity, this text focuses on key hospital processes and IT applications; however, parallel concepts in other healthcare venues, such as long-term care and home health care, and both large and small medical group practices, are incorporated, typically as additional examples or case studies.

This book explains how improved quality of patient-centric care ultimately increases productivity and key relationships between quality and productivity. This critical relationship is reiterated by describing how quality drivers increase competitiveness, lower costs, and enhance long-term organizational viability. Although unique in both content and approach, this textbook links quality and productivity by illustrating how these essential objectives of patient-centric care delivery are achieved.

Examples and illustrations of tools and techniques and how they are commonly used by multidisciplinary cross-functional teams to improve quality and productivity are included. Quality concepts incorporate philosophies from experts like Deming, Juran, Ishikawa, Crosby, Labowitz, and Caldwell.

This book presents a transformation strategy in the context of three critical and interconnected components: quality, productivity, and technology management. Links among these components are preserved throughout the book. Healthcare executives, managers, supervisors, management engineers, clinicians, and others will benefit as traditional IT needs of students in health administration are addressed. Never before has there been such intense emphasis and open debate in the healthcare industry about improving quality and patient focus and critical safety issues throughout healthcare delivery processes.

This primer provides the necessary context, tools, and techniques to prepare aspiring transformationalists to lead technology-driven "order of magnitude" improvement.

CHAPTER 1

Digitally Transforming Health Care: An Introduction

This chapter introduces strategies for digital transformation of health care, justifies the need for this book, and, most importantly, describes an approach that drives effective change into a patient-centric seamlessly integrated network that delivers high-quality, efficient, and effective health care.

Key Concepts

- Rationale and analytic strategies, textbook structure, and organization
- Organization and intended learning structure with chapter highlights
- Multidisciplinary need for an integrated, patient-centric, digital transformation of healthcare delivery

---

INTRODUCTION

A heightened level of awareness and special interest by payers, employers, and healthcare processionals has been driven by the exponential rise in healthcare delivery costs during the last decade. Society has for some time recognized that this unsustainable trend reflects an urgent need for a dramatic increase in quality and competitiveness. More recently, this recognition has been coupled with an amplified awareness of much more consumer-oriented patients, employers, and payers who have now driven health care to the very top of America's political agenda. A number of states have legislated mandatory healthcare insurance coverage for residents and more states are in the process of creating similar legislature. The days of uncontrolled and unlimited healthcare resource consumption are history. Increasingly competitive pressure has forced leaders to recognize that radical processes redesign to rapidly streamline operations is long overdue, and without focused effective action providers will quickly become uncompetitive and risk organizational irrelevance. All stakeholders in the healthcare industry are experiencing these demands for reform, forcing fundamental organizational change, a new technologic philosophy, and an urgency for significantly improved performance.

This digital transformation began with federal regulations. Now all providers must be deliberately focused to simultaneously ensure patient safety, significantly increase quality, and substantially reduce costs as mandated rather than as just desirable objectives. This transformation cannot be based solely on a definition of quality from the Joint Commission on Accreditation of Healthcare Organizations (JCAHO). This pervasive patient-centric transformation must be driven by customer's needs, wants, and expectations.

What is urgently needed is a visible affirmation of leadership's commitment to pursue quality as a vital mission of the organization. Quality is not just a socially provocative idea. Quality and cost are two key criteria by which employer, payers, and patients now evaluate healthcare purchase decisions. Quality has become a key strategic element of healthcare management in response to these very well-informed consumers. Any healthcare organization that is not focusing in a patient-centric manner on internal and external customers is writing a prescription for failure. A dramatic paradigm shift has occurred as patients have become more knowledgeable and now behave as assertive customers with demanding expectations. These behaviors must be effectively integrated into clinical processes and care delivery service designs. This paradigm shift represents a fundamental "sea change" from traditional provider behaviors that were guided by a notion that providers know best.

In response to these demanding challenges, providers now recognize that an effective transformational response must be driven by aggressive business strategy. Such an approach relies on digital transformation as leverage to consistently deliver safer higher quality patient care with increasing operational effectiveness and improved productivity. Such a savvy strategy requires a substantial IT investment that results in comprehensively redesigned "mission critical" processes. Today, progressive digitally transformed provider organizations have already gone beyond advanced clinical systems with the early adoption of seamlessly integrated information and medical technologies, requiring substantial process redesign in all care delivery venues throughout every organization.

Traditional healthcare organizations have long been criticized for extended retention of outdated legacy systems, resisting adoption of decidedly disruptive and contemporary transformational technologies that require rigorous process redesign. By continuing this reactive posture and deferring inevitable acquisition and adoption of more effective patient-centric transformational technologies to improve care delivery safety, quality, and efficiency, these organizations are lagging further and further behind more digitally adaptive organizations. Competition is already leveraging transformational technologies. These "disruptive technologies" are pervasive and seamlessly integrate communications, imaging, and information among and between diagnostic centers, laboratories, patient care venues, pharmacies, surgical suites, nurse call and communications systems, lighting systems, pagers, cellular and mobile phones, personal digital assistants (PDAs), and heating, ventilating, and air conditioning (HVAC) systems.

HISTORICAL PERSPECTIVES

Digitally transformed pioneers have simplified, streamlined, and redesigned processes to increase and expedite throughput with compressed delivery cycle times to adapt to increasingly demanding market forces. These pace-setting provider organizations produce and consume real-time information to expedite and improve care delivery with updated clinical data as demanded by both quality-driven physicians and assertive patients empowered with information. Additionally, these pioneers have an improved capability to generate quality data to meet payer's increasing demands and to prepare for inevitable reimbursement changes as they occur.

Transformational information technologies digitize current technology and instruments on seamlessly integrated data networks to enable real-time clinician access into each patient's longitudinal electronic medical record (EMR), anytime, anywhere. Digitally advanced hospitals have demonstrated reduced lengths of stay, increased care quality, and increased reimbursement that generates generous margins. Quantitative benefits are incremental and sometimes challenging to realize and even more difficult to credibly demonstrate measurable material return on significant upfront investments. Pioneering providers who made these investments in transformational technologies (i.e., at least 5% or more of operating budgets) have achieved and can enjoy these digitized capabilities.

Early initiatives in digital transformation with computing in health care can be traced back more than 50 years when only mainframe computers were available and only in major hospitals with sufficient resources (i.e., funding, time, and effort) to afford to acquire, install, house, maintain, and use these machines. Examples of these early pioneers are

- El Camino Hospital, Mountain View, California
- Monmouth Medical Center, Long Branch, New Jersey

- Veteran's Administration, Washington, DC
- Danderyd Hospital, Stockholm, Sweden
- London Hospital, London, England
- Hanover Hospital, Hanover, Germany

Hardware and software vendors and system integrators, all with reputations for effective design, project management, and implementation of complex systems in other service industries, joined with these hospitals to collaborate, develop, and support very early versions of patient information systems. Examples of vendors who demonstrated visionary insight for market opportunities are

- Burroughs Corporation
- Control Data Corporation
- General Electric
- Honeywell, Inc.
- International Business Machines (IBM)
- National Cash Register Company (NCR)
- Lockheed Information Systems Division
- McDonnell-Douglas
- Technicon Corporation

No single vendor, system, or application can be considered representative of all others because of different needs, goals, and anticipated impacts in each provider organization. For example, unique requirements for design and infrastructure, functions and features, and variable technical and technology investment capabilities had to be customized in each development site. That said, for historical perspective a case study is presented on the now legendary experiences at El Camino Hospital in Mountain View, California.

CASE STUDY

This facility has been selected for this case study because of its operational experience with a broad range of IT and evolutionary care delivery changes that have occurred over time. This organization's experiences are reflective of early healthcare information system (HIS) development initiatives and system capabilities that were representative HIS prototypes, characteristics, and rich functions and features for more than 50 years.

System development at El Camino Hospital began as a successful pioneering prototype that was widely recognized as an effective model for healthcare digital transformation for ongoing development of patient information management systems throughout North America and Europe. Lessons learned during this project focused on user information needs and requirements to change skeptical physician and nurse user attitudes. Similar experiences could be described for other provider organizations and a variety of commercially available healthcare IT applications with similar rich histories.

When this prototype system was installed, El Camino was a 450-bed community general hospital with a medical staff of 340 physicians, serving patients under the care of personal physicians (i.e., a nonteaching hospital without any internship or residency program). At that time the hospital provided emergency room care and diagnostic procedures for patients referred by staff physicians. Various versions and upgrades to hardware and software supported the operation at El Camino Hospital since 1972. Three years of system development at the hospital preceded initial prototype implementation. Installation of this initial system version throughout the hospital took 9 months, after which the National Center for Health Services Research awarded funds to El Camino Hospital for evaluation of the project. System hardware, a large mainframe computer, was located at a regional computer center several miles from El Camino Hospital, with a second computer available for backup support. Data were maintained at this central processing facility using magnetic disks and reel-to-reel tapes for temporary and archival storage.

El Camino Hospital's 58 video terminals and 31 printers were linked to this computer center via dedicated high-speed telephone lines. Most software was written in assembly language, using COBOL for financial reports. This prototype system was a true hospital-wide system designed to store patient and financial data and to aggregate and communicate appropriate data and information, either automatically or upon request.

Hospital objectives for this first-generation patient care information system included provision of

- More efficient healthcare delivery
- Improved patient care by facilitating and enhancing nursing and ancillary department activities
- Reduction and/or containment of operational costs

Physicians, nurses, ancillary service personnel, and admitting staff entered data through video terminals, which consisted of a light video sensitive screen, keyboard, and light pen for rapid selection of information presented on the screen. *Direct physician use,* which has historically distinguished this system from most other hospital-wide systems then and now, requires nursing or other support personnel to enter data for physicians. Terminals were located at each nursing station and in ancillary service departments. Authorized personnel accessed the system by typing a unique user identification code on the keyboard. This security procedure ensured that hospital personnel could only enter, change, view, and print information relevant to their job.

As a terminal screen displayed a list of items (e.g., laboratory tests that a physician desired to order), a specific item was selected and entered into the computer system by pointing a light pen at the desired phrase and pressing a switch on the barrel of the pen. Using this light pen, a physician could enter a full set of medical orders (e.g., laboratory work, medications, x-rays, diet, activity, etc.) for a specific patient.

These displays reminded physicians to make complete orders; for example, when a medication was ordered, the display noted the need to specify scheduling and method of administration (i.e., oral, intravenous, or intramuscular) in addition to dosage. The keyboard was used to enter any information that was not displayed on the video display. A physician or nurse at the nursing station printed copies of orders for verification and then these verified orders were automatically routed and printed in each appropriate ancillary department for diagnostic or therapeutic service.

This successful demonstration project led to other large-scale data processing applications in medicine and health record systems as computer growth accelerated in other industries. Hospitals began to justify additional system investment and then demonstrate continuing productivity gains and early evidence of increased process efficiency.

These early successes were achieved at very high costs, emphasizing the need for senior executive leadership to take responsibility for organizational transformation (e.g., anticipate and prepare for resistance from some staff). Approximately 10% of user personnel were adaptive and embraced these operational changes rather quickly. Another 10 to 15% demonstrated passive resistance to changes and eventually left the organization because of their inability to effectively adapt to transformation-related process changes throughout the organization. Others eventually adapted as required by emulating behavior changes of earlier adapters.

El Camino Hospital continues to use this industry-leading technical platform to support an effective, efficient, and rich portfolio of state-of-the-art functions and features that have facilitated and sustained digital transformation for more than 50 years. Over time, this initially mainframe-based system has been upgraded and is now integrating unique intelligence gathering via an Internet protocol (IP)-based network infrastructure with knowledge-driven clinical, financial, and management information software and services throughout the enterprise. As recently as 2005, El Camino Hospital has continued to be repeatedly named to the Honor Roll of the *U.S. News & World Report* annual "America's Best Hospitals List."

A number of these Honor Roll hospitals use this system vendor's clinical applications, including the perennially top-ranked facility, The Johns Hopkins Hospital. Most of these "digitally transformed" providers use integrated clinical decision support, informatics, and computerized physician order entry (CPOE) applications to enable managers to effectively provide safe, efficient, and accurate patient care as well as to analyze and manage operations.

Keystone Systems, the healthcare industry's recognized information system benchmarking report, indicates that this vendor's CPOE solutions are in use by more inpatient organizations and by more physicians than CPOE solutions from all other vendors. Keystone Systems is an independent research and consulting firm that specializes in monitoring and reporting performance of healthcare IT vendors and healthcare professional services firms.

This vendor has been repeatedly recognized as a leading provider of solutions based on physician usage in the Keystone Systems' *CPOE Digest 2005*, which reported that when ease-of-use and rich functional capabilities are key decision-making criterion, healthcare organizations selected this system more often than other vendor. Interoperability of this system's applications represents an important digital transformation achievement by El Camino Hospital and other provider organization users as required to achieve the U.S. federal government's goal of a nationwide EMR for most Americans by 2014.

Having been recognized worldwide as an industry leader in remote healthcare information processing and having met rigorous standards and requirements of the ISO 9001:2000 certification program, this systems integrator has been registered as an ISO 9001:2000-compliant company. Microsoft Corporation and this vendor recently announced a multiple year strategic alliance.

With a single clinical platform spanning an entire healthcare enterprise and linking these applications to the community, this system received InfoWorld's Top 100 Award for 2005 as one of the most innovative uses of enterprise technology in health care. This award was given for an interoperative wireless companion to all advanced clinical solutions, enabling wireless access to real-time clinical data anytime from anywhere.

MODERN DEVELOPMENTS

Today, a digital hospital relies on technology as an integral and fundamental part of business strategy. Technology is applied to every facet of clinical and business operations, such as integrating patients, personnel, process, technology, and cultural elements. IT is now defined more broadly as healthcare providers go beyond advanced clinical systems to include fundamental patient-centric integration and digital transformation of strategic processes associated with information and medical technologies. Industry standards and legislation, such as the Health Insurance Portability and Accountability Act (HIPAA) and the Clinical Context Object Workgroup (CCOW), are leveraging seamless connectivity to enhance more effective communication among stakeholders and business partners in the community.

There are an increasing number of real-world examples that innovative providers recognize and embrace requirements that are best achieved through IT-driven digital transformation. Organizations described as digital hospitals tend to be stand-alone, newly built, specialty facilities designed as advanced highly automated facilities. Digital value was embraced in initial designs of these facilities. Fundamental principles driving digital transformation within any healthcare provider organization have been emulated from successful automation experiences in healthcare and other service industries.

As of this writing, specific goals associated with digital transformation have yet to be clearly articulated because a comprehensive vision of future health and healthcare delivery has not yet coalesced. Most community hospitals have at least some automation of patient registration, scheduling, and billing as well as within laboratories, imaging, and pharmacy departments.

Governmental leadership at the federal, state, and regional level is being coordinated by an increasing number of collaborative initiatives that focus on specific components of a truly standardized national infrastructure required to achieve a functional EMR in all delivery venues a reality. Examples of these collaborations are as follows:

- Workgroup for Electronic Data Interchange-Strategic National Implementation Process (WEDI-SNIP) is a nonprofit organization dedicated to improving health care through support of national and regional electronic commerce initiatives.
- Typical programs, conferences, policy, and advisory white papers have included
  - HIPAA Strategic National Implementation Process
  - National Provider Identifier Outreach Initiative
  - WEDI Regional Affiliates Academic Medical Centers Events Groups
  - Clinical and Electronic Health Record Initiatives
- WEDI members and other healthcare stakeholders have been informed and educated about benefits and strategies to improve information management and exchange.
- As a leading advisory group to the Centers for Medicare and Medicare (CMS) in the Department of Health and Human Services (DHHS), WEDI-SNIP facilitated national and regional collaboration, providing policy guid-

ance and leadership to the healthcare industry on how to use and leverage the industry's collective knowledge, expertise, and information resources to improve the quality, affordability, and availability of health care. For example, WEDI-SNIP was the leading policy advisory organization to CMS administrators during regulatory development and implementation phases of HIPAA Title II, a massive conversion of healthcare electric data exchange privacy and security regulations.

- The College of Healthcare Information Management Executives (CHIME) provides professional development programs and services exclusively for CIOs in health care. CHIME advocates more effective use of information management within health care. CHIME events and activities were designed to reflect these objectives (e.g., CIO-oriented surveys, benchmarking data on staffing ratios, sample documents, job descriptions, research, education forums, focus groups, and peer networking activities).

Recent advances in information systems, networks, and telecommunication technologies enable global real-time collaboration and consultation among and between physicians and other members of the healthcare delivery team. As an example, therapeutic remote monitoring and robotic surgical procedures are increasingly common. These interactions are conducted via secure networks that provide sufficient bandwidth to support simultaneous voice, data, images, and text.

Healthcare professionals are challenged to embrace each technological advance, thereby requiring lifelong learning. Digital transformationalists must continually gain and sustain state-of-the-art knowledge, acquire necessary skills, and develop and demonstrate expertise and technical competency. Providers in all venues are continually challenged to deliver higher quality lower cost patient care while using fewer and less-expensive resources. Organizational viability of current providers can only be sustained by achieving higher levels of productivity at all levels. Within the last decade medical technology has advanced more than in the last 100 years. As clinical information accumulates with instantaneous access and at an ever-increasing rate, healthcare professionals are challenged to process and use information about new discoveries, medications, procedures, and technology even before these products and services are commercially available.

As technology is changing lives, ethical considerations and choices associated with breakthrough applications of this technology are having varied and far-reaching implications. Currently, IT professionals are discovering, designing, implementing, and using these applications and will be introducing, experiencing, and assessing benefits of these new and continually emerging technologies early in their careers. Today's aspiring healthcare professionals need to be aware of this awesome responsibility and the multitude of difficult choices awaiting them.

A broad definition of computer and systems literacy is necessary to begin to understand how to rapidly acquire and aggregate these data and then instantly present accurate and meaningful information to authorized personnel. Hence, some working definitions are presented:

- A **computer** is an electronic device capable of rapidly and reliably enabling data input and performing manipulation, storage, calculation, communication, informational transformation, reporting, and presentation.
- **Information systems** are a group of interoperable components, applications, and associated technologies working together to complete a set of specified tasks.

This book is an examination of applications supporting a variety of clinicians and many other healthcare professionals with varying degrees of computer knowledge and proficiency. Hospital and other provider organizations are beginning and will have to then sustain a digital transformation that becomes increasingly automated with ever-more sophisticated systems and telecommunication networks. As this technical evolution advances, providers are increasingly dependent on IT to manage workflow and perform work by an increasing computer-literate workforce.

IT professionals, systems and operations analysts, and management engineers must be more knowledgeable about computers and related terminology to be capable of explaining their use and competently designing, developing, acquiring, implementing, maintaining, and refining systems, applications, and associated processes and tasks. IT literate professionals must be aware of social and ethical questions concerning computers and information systems and associated transformational applications, processes, and tasks. Although IT provides many benefits to our society, misuse and abuse of computer technology can and does occur.

CHAPTER 2

Multi-disciplinary Concepts: A Fundamental Foundation

This chapter introduces data collection topics, analytic techniques, and team dynamics tools. These essential tools and techniques are used to collect, aggregate, and analyze data. When used in various combinations, these techniques generate team discussions that lead to effective decision-making by team consensus. Examples of these techniques and concepts are

- Brainstorming
- Flowcharting and "imagineering"
- Force field analysis
- Ishikawa (or cause and effect) diagramming
- Nominal group techniques (NGTs)
- Pareto analysis
- Run and control charting

The initial focus is on common tools used by process improvement teams, business process reengineering task forces, and IT professionals of all disciplines. All IT professionals must be proficient to effectively lead digital transformation initiatives in health care. As digital transformationalists, these multidisciplinary individuals lead process redesign and automation-driven projects using a variety of ITs.

FLOWCHART

A flowchart is a fundamental tool used to explain, communicate, and facilitate a collaborative understanding of a process, including logic and essential relationships among and between various process or system components. Flowcharts document how systems, applications, functions, and processes operate. This graphic tool is sometimes considered to be an "imagineering" tool that visualizes and facilitates analyses to identify problems, bottlenecks, delays, and opportunities for potential process improvements. Analysts can visualize each unique component, task, decision, and event in a process to understand their relationships to design, reengineer, or imagine an "ideal" process. Visual images are easier to understand and explain than painstaking descriptions of the same process documented in lengthy paragraphs or narrative pages.

> A flowchart is a graphic representation of a process enabling teams and team members to better visualize and understand key operational sequences, decisions, delays, movements, and storage activities within a process or system.

Truly, a picture is worth a thousand words. Team members from different disciplines can quickly understand key functions, decisions, and relationships in a process. A flowchart has defined start and end points to establish boundaries and to frame each perspective for analysis. Typical events such as answering a telephone call, taking a patient's vital signs, and printing orders are each functional components that constitute a process and as such are depicted in a process flowchart. Each event is represented by a symbol that has a distinct meaning and is connected by arrows indicating both direction and logic of process flow with a distinct end point. Process flowchart construction requires discussion and collaboration of knowledgeable team members who are stakeholders of each portion for the entire process and who are recognized as "subject matter experts" regarding each key process component.

Flowchart construction requires a team to

- *Define* start and end points and identify key workflow components, decisions points, and related flowchart steps
- *Collaborate* and *document* each process step and thereby enable all team members and executive sponsors to review and understand process beginning and ending points
- *Define* and *document* assumptions to avoid any potential confusion
- *Sequence* each process, task, or event

- *Assign* a symbol, such as those in Figure 2.1
- *Validate* this clearly and concisely developed process flow with personnel involved in the process and most knowledgeable about each relevant process component
- *Identify* and *correct* any gaps to eliminate any misunderstandings

Process automation technologists and digital transformationalists use variations of these simple generic flowchart symbols to depict unique activities or actions. Many variations and additional symbols are used. Symbols are occasionally customized as necessary to show unique characteristics that are dependent on each process, or system, as well as to explain specialized activities.

Historically, systems analysts and computer programmers used flowcharts to graphically document logical and detailed steps encoded in computer programs. Operations analysts, management engineers, and process improvement, reengineering, and Six Sigma teams commonly use flowcharts to document current states and depict future states of processes or systems under study. This aspect of flowcharting and process documentation is vital to ensure that all team members understand complete processes or workflows, even though individual team members may have expert knowledge of only a limited portion of an entire process.

Figure 2.2 illustrates a simple process flowchart depicting outpatient clinic visit process activities from beginning to end. Figure 2.3 is an example of a "deployment"

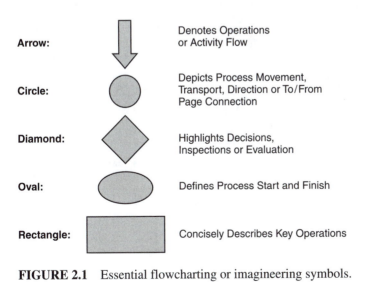

FIGURE 2.1   Essential flowcharting or imagineering symbols.

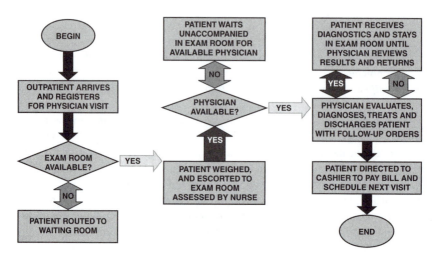

FIGURE 2.2   Process flowchart documenting current state of outpatient clinic visit process.

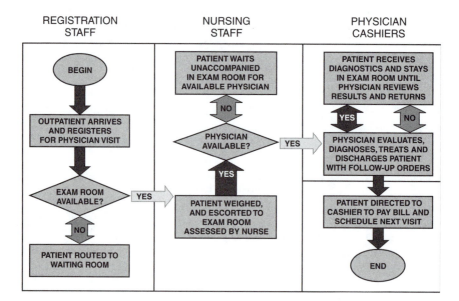

FIGURE 2.3   Example of horizontal or deployment flowchart.

or "horizontal" flowchart showing process actions by different individuals or departments. This variation is frequently used to show complex process "hand-offs" from individual to individual or from department to department. These hand-off transactions are very often opportunities for process improvement. Many commercial, open source, and software programs include capabilities to quickly and accurately develop flowcharts of many types and to edit with corrections and changes over time.

PARETO CHARTING AND ANALYSIS

Pareto analyses facilitate data organization and presentation to isolate and show those "vital few causes" of a problem from the "trivial many."

Pareto Principle: 80/20 Rule

Pareto developed the "80/20 rule": 80% of problems are caused by 20% of personnel.

Pareto charts are the most widely and creatively used process improvement tools. Pareto analyses facilitate data organization and presentation to isolate and show those "vital few causes" of a problem from the "trivial many." This technique is best used when problems must be identified to focus team members on a relevant issue and further isolate and eliminate others from consideration and analysis. Team efforts can then effectively focus on those problems, offering the most potential for substantial process or system improvement. A Pareto diagram displays the relative frequency or size in either an ascending or descending bar graph. Ideally suited to focus team attention on key problems, this tool is especially useful to identify opportunities of a highest value. Quality improvement, process reengineering, or a Six Sigma team can effectively allocate resources by using the Pareto technique to do the following:

- *Understand* relative importance of problems in a simple, quickly interpreted, visual format
- *Reduce* the probability of shifting a problem because a proposed solution removes some causes but worsens others (i.e., the result of unintended consequences; there is no net organizational benefit by simply moving a problem from one department to another)
- *Measure* progress using a visible and easy to understand format

As depicted in Figure 2.4, a Pareto diagram construction involves

- *Identifying* problems to be investigated
- *Collecting* appropriate data and using Pareto analysis techniques to analyze zero-based data types (e.g., a number of complaints with an expectation that an ideal situation will reduce complaints to zero)
- *Classifying* data by categories such as type of complaints, nursing units or departments, shifts, diagnosis-related groups (DRGs), and patients
- *Arranging* error categories by type, quantity, and percentage in either ascending or descending order
- *Stratifying* data as required (i.e., weekly data grouped into weekdays and weekends and then classified by day or by shift as subgroups based on unique characteristics or useful categories)
- *Creating* Pareto diagrams as specialized bar graphs (e.g., displaying types of patient complaints, their respective totals, percentage of overall total, cumulative totals, and cumulative percentages)
- *Drawing* a cumulative Pareto curve with cumulative percentages above interval (e.g., each complaint connected with a solid line)
- *Verifying* that each graph displays an obvious Pareto pattern (i.e., categories with similar percentages may require an alternative stratification of data so that distinct problem categories are isolated)

For example, as depicted in Figure 2.4, patient complaints should be categorized, with infrequent complaints included as an "all others" category. If an "all

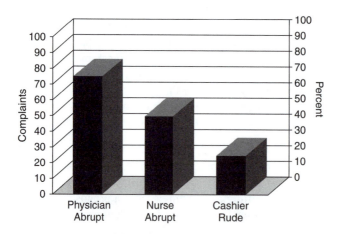

FIGURE 2.4   Pareto analysis: patient perceptions of emergency staff attitudes.

others" bar reflects more than 50% of the largest individual bar in the graph, the "all others" category should be separated and then displayed individually.

Pareto analysis and interpretation focuses on the tallest bars first because those categories usually represent major contributing causes to the problem under study. Focusing on these problem categories first results in more expeditious problem-solving and deploys scarce resources most effectively.

Pareto graph construction, display, and analysis must include perceptions of patients, staff, and other key stakeholders in any process being studied. As with most tools, there are a number of specialized variations. For example, variations of Pareto diagrams include "cause" breakdowns as tallest bars are broken into sub-causes in subsequently linked Pareto diagrams. This limited overview highlights the typical presentation that is most useful in multidisciplinary team initiatives.

ISHIKAWA (CAUSE AND EFFECT) DIAGRAMMING

Ishikawa diagramming is a common technique used for initial problem identification and dispersion analysis. A team's learning curve through these incremental steps is necessary to discover each critical problem in a process and to understand each problem's root cause(s).

> An Ishikawa, or cause and effect, diagram enables a team to identify, isolate, explore, and display each cause in increasing detail while demonstrating an understanding of all possible causes related to a problem or condition.

By using Ishikawa diagramming techniques, digital transformation teams focus on problems, not on various symptoms or other distractions, differing interests, or unique and sometimes important disciplinary bias. This analysis encourages all team members to gain a consistent collective knowledge about a problem and to develop team consensus and support for further analyses of potential solutions. A classic Ishikawa diagram resembles a fish skeleton with causes presented as vertebrae branching from a central spine that leads to an observable effect. As depicted in Figure 2.5, initial versions of an Ishikawa diagram usually take a generic form of a fish skeleton with branches (vertebrae) shown as core policies, personnel, processes, and procedures or people, methods, material, instruments, and equipment. Additional team consideration, discussion, and brainstorming yield increasingly detailed breakdowns of these causes. Ultimately, a root cause or causes are presented as vertebrae, frequently requiring further data collection and validation using other tools.

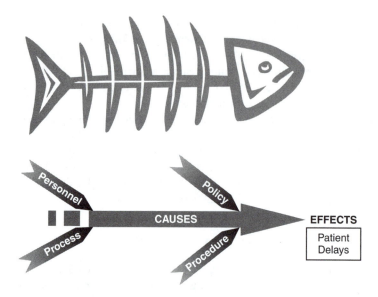

FIGURE 2.5   Ishikawa (fishbone) or cause and effect diagram.

Ishikawa developed and applied this tool to early quality analysis of factory processes studied by Deming in Japan.

Typically, an Ishikawa diagram is used after likely causes are identified by using other tools, such as flowcharting, brainstorming, NGT, or Pareto analysis. Actual construction of an Ishikawa diagram is the most elemental of its use. Analysis differentiates true causes from symptoms of a problem. Identified causes are then further analyzed with other techniques or tools to understand relationships among and between causes while exploring opportunities for process improvement. This tool is also used to document and track changes in patterns or observed deviations from previously anticipated norms or expected effects.

A *dispersion analysis* is developed as an Ishikawa diagram is constructed by placing individual causes within each "major" cause category and then asking about each individual cause with questions like, "Why does this cause (dispersion) happen?" These questions are repeated for each level of detail until potential causes are exhausted. Use of this simple "why" technique, is espoused by Labovitz et al.

This technique is most effective when sequentially exploring through at least three response levels and then displaying responses as more detailed branches off each major cause. Further interpretation is necessary to discover underlying issues and to develop a credible consensus that identifies a root cause for each problem (a fundamental underlying cause). Causes that appear repeatedly may require more data to determine relative frequencies of each cause and ultimately to discover a root cause. When this root cause is eliminated or effectively modified, a "future state" solution is presented. This graphic presentation is very effective when describing a before and after picture of problem resolution.

RUN CHARTS

Run charts show trends as observations over time. They are used to visualize process characteristics such as errors and increased or decreased activity that changes over time. Meaningful trends can be identified as a team monitors unusual events in a process that affects average process performance. This basic tool enables team members to visualize individual data points and to monitor a process to see if a "trend" is developing or changing.

> Run charts highlight process changes and variations as a team plots and studies observations. Data points are plotted in sequence when available.

Run charts are simple to construct and easy to use and interpret. As with other charting techniques, team members should focus only on critical changes, being cautious not to consider every variation as significant. Teams use run charts to monitor performance and identify meaningful trends or shifts in average process performances.

In clinical laboratories, known control specimens are included in each "run" of glucose analyses to ensure that all reagents and instrument components are performing within expected specifications. Figure 2.6 is a run chart showing control values for a month. Because control chart construction begins with an overlay of a run chart with statistical control protocols, this data set is also used in control chart examples:

- *Track* useful information.
- *Predict* potential variation as data are collected and plotted.
- *Focus* attention on vital changes to detect meaningful trends.

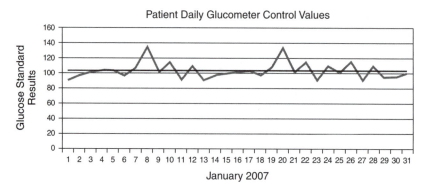

FIGURE 2.6   Example of a run chart.

* *If favorable*, a change should be evaluated and considered a potential process improvement.
* *If unfavorable*, team members must consider countermeasures that reduce unfavorable process variation.

CONTROL CHARTS

Control charts are graphs that display process characteristics and compare process performance with statistically derived control limits that measure process variation. Understanding and mastering run chart concepts, construction, and use to identify process variation is necessary before moving on with this natural transition to even more fundamental statistical process principles. These concepts and traditional industrial engineering principles have evolved from their manufacturing origins.

> Control charts show that a process *is or is not* in "statistical control" and to determine whether a statistically controlled process can be maintained.

Deming developed these principles to understand and measure process variation over time. By constructing and using control charts with control limits, IT professionals can incorporate IT to monitor and manage any healthcare delivery process. Deming concluded that quality is best achieved by simply controlling and managing process variation. Similarly, radical improvement of care delivery processes is more effectively attained by applying robust IT applications to drive digital transformation of mission critical processes.

All processes exhibit some inherent variation because variation is simply unavoidable. For example, an expected proportion of laboratory analytic or billing errors varies from one day to another. By recognizing this information as fundamental fact, a conscientious effort is made to control and reduce variation. Common cause variations are due to variations that are inherent in a process. Special cause variations are not inherent in a process but are controllable by management:

- Poor workplace lighting or other aspects of a worker's environment
- Ill-equipped tools, excessive background noise, and poor ventilation
- Instrumentation or other equipment malfunction
- Poorly designed technical tools, software interfaces, or information systems
- Management failure to provide feedback to each worker

All variation is due to either common or special causes.

Although complex statistical and comprehensive quantitative analyses are sometimes difficult to understand and master, they are fundamental concepts and metrics commonly used to manage healthcare delivery process performance by decreasing process variance from average performance:

- A *control limit* is a line (or lines) on a control chart used to assess process variation significance.
- *Variation* is the difference of output values of a process from the process mean.
  - Variation reflects *both* common causes and special causes. Variation beyond a control limit reflects special causes affecting a process.
  - Graphic problem-solving techniques (e.g., control charts) display these variations as important "current state" problems to be solved and show whether "future state" interventions have been effective enough to demonstrate a sustainable and controlled process.
- *Statistical process control* uses statistical tools and techniques (e.g., control charts) to analyze process capability, outputs, or outcomes. Appropriate management action or other necessary countermeasures are required to achieve and sustain improved process capability.
- *Data universe* is a population under study from which a sample is drawn.
- *Prevention* is a future-oriented strategy that improves quality by directing analysis and action to correct processes, not ad-hoc problems. Prevention

reflects a philosophy of continuous improvement demonstrated by less process variation over time.

- *Value distribution* around a process's mean performance patterns is consistent with concepts implying that anything measured repeatedly will produce different results.
- *Observations* of process outputs and outcomes occur in statistically predictable patterns and have been associated with the "Hawthorne effect" by some experts.

A normal distribution of these data points results in a classic bell-shaped curve with most observations near the process mean, with fewer and fewer observations falling evenly on either side of this process average. Figure 2.7 and Figure 2.8 show this conceptual construct and depict classic bell curves being transformed into a control chart. This transformation shows the mean and each standard deviation of a bell curve becoming control limits on a control chart. This fundamental process improvement tool and technique were derived from a traditional "central tendency theorem" and related statistical control theory to discover, understand, and quantify the variability of a process's current state.

QM, continuous process improvement, process reengineering, and Six Sigma teams use control charts to analyze problem causes. After reviewing this information the team can develop the comprehensive understanding necessary to formulate consensus, present an effective solution, and execute their solution using a corrective countermeasure or action plan. After implementation the team continues to monitor process performance using control charts to sustain improved statistical process control over time.

As introduced earlier, a control chart is a run chart with a statistically derived upper control limit (UCL) and lower control limit (LCL). These control limits are

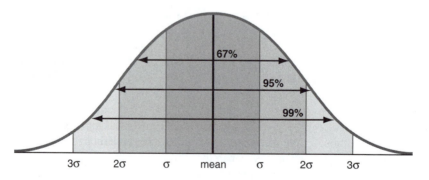

FIGURE 2.7   Bell curve with 1, 2, and 3 standard deviations.

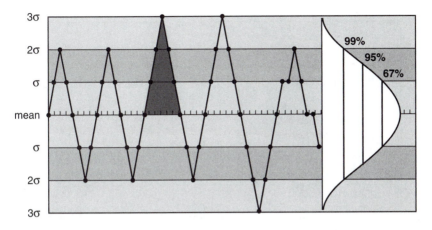

FIGURE 2.8   Normal bell curve transformation.

displayed as horizontal lines on either side of a process's arithmetic average on the chart's *x*-axis. Data points are individual values of process performance criteria used to determine whether a process is "under statistical process control." Usually, a sample size of 20 to 30 variables is drawn from a dynamic database and collected during a predetermined time frame. Variability of these values is used to statistically calculate UCLs and LCLs. Control limits reflect process capability compared with predetermined specifications and should *not* be confused with a patient's wants, needs, requirements, or expectations.

> A process may be in control but not capable of producing outputs or outcomes that meet required specifications.
>
> "In control" does *not* imply that process outputs or outcomes meet system needs or patient expectations. This technique is a metric used to express process consistency (i.e., either consistently acceptable or consistently unacceptable).

Variation beyond control limit represents special causes affecting a process. Graphic problem-solving techniques (e.g., control charts) display these variations as important problems to be solved and show that interventions have been effective enough to produce a controlled process. Some variation is random or otherwise due to unique characteristics of a process that is in statistical control.

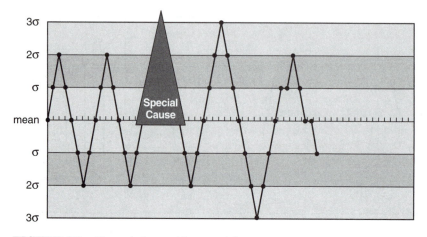

FIGURE 2.9   Control chart with a special cause.

UCLs and LCLs at 1, 2, and 3 standard deviations are determined and displayed above and below the arithmetic mean of a process control chart. Figure 2.9 shows special cause variation as shaded data points above the UCL. Fluctuations within control limits represent variation that is inherent to a process. Common causes within a process or system (e.g., inadequate design, equipment limitations, outdated policy or historical protocols, incorrect operating procedures, inadequate preventive maintenance) are affected by a system or process change. Values outside of control limits represent special causes (e.g., personnel error(s), unplanned events, unusual accidents or occurrences, unintended circumstances) that are not characteristic of a typical process in operation. Special causes must be addressed by management to be corrected, modified, or eliminated before a control chart will accurately depict that a process is "in control" when operating and monitored on an ongoing basis. After a process has demonstrated that consistently in control outputs or outcomes are produced and ongoing monitoring confirms that no fundamental change has occurred, then and only then can a process be considered as "in statistical control."

Senior management must actively support opportunities to control and reduce variation in key organizational processes and systems. Such initiative support is needed during development and execution, requiring necessary intervention, and then again after an intervention, demonstrating an effectively transformed process by requiring necessary monitoring to ensure sustainable change.

During this process team members and executive sponsors should encourage questions to gain an understanding from both a process behavior and a statistical process control perspective:

- Are there differences in measuring instrument accuracy used?
- Are there differences in methods used by different staff members?
- Is process affected by varying environmental or organizational factors (e.g., temperature, humidity, budgetary constraints, staffing, scheduling)?
- Has there been a significant environmental or organizational change?
- Were any untrained staff members, students, or interns involved?
- Have supply sources changed?
- Could staff fatigue affect this process?
- Has there been a change in maintenance procedures?
- How are instruments changed or adjusted?
- Did errors occur with different instruments or equipment, shifts, or operators?
- Are staff members reluctant to report "bad news"?

Staff should *not* be held responsible for problems that are due to common variations. Management must accept responsibility to resolve common causes of variation.

Special cause variations are due to events outside process or system control limits.

Special cause variations are typically avoidable and cannot be overlooked (e.g., cases caused by not following certain prescribed standards or improper application of standards). Special causes are frequently associated with differences among workers, methods, or instruments. Both common and special cause variations should be identified and managed. When variations are due to special causes, a presence of certain meaningful factors is implied and should be investigated.

Another control chart should be prepared after process improvement or after corrective countermeasures have been implemented. This control chart displays a "future state" as experienced, indicating whether or not these interventions were adequate enough to bring this process under control. For mission critical processes, even processes under control may still be so broken that continuous process improvement or business process reengineering projects will not produce acceptable outcomes. These situations are best addressed in conjunction with Six Sigma initiatives, as described in Chapter 12.

Figure 2.10 reflects a process brought under control as demonstrated by control charts. Control charts are developed from run charts and are routinely used in a clinical laboratory to monitor patient glucose analyses. A "before" control chart identified unacceptable special cause variation (Figure 2.10, Out of Control

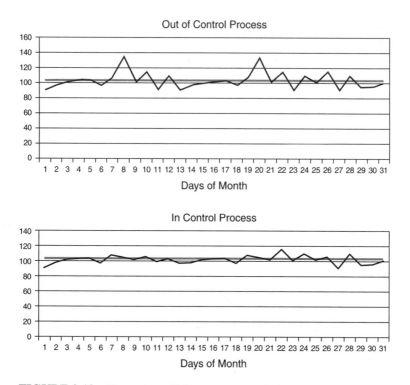

FIGURE 2.10   Examples of laboratory control charts.

Process, top). This graph reflects an out of control analysis because not all plotted points are within control limits. After investigation the laboratory manager determined that the cause of a variation was in fact special, and steps were immediately taken to permanently eliminate the cause. Revised policies and procedures were developed and staff were retrained to prevent a recurrence.

The control chart shown at the bottom of Figure 2.10 (In Control Process) shows this process after special causes of variation have been eliminated. After investigation and procedure changes were made to eliminate these special causes, no "out-of-control" values were experienced. Several such iterations may be needed to stabilize a process and bring it under control as determined to meet management requirements.

Table 2.1 summarizes the most common technical types of control charts used in healthcare process reengineering and digital transformation initiatives. Each type of control chart is listed in decreasing order of common use, including a typ-

TABLE 2.1   Control Chart Types

Type	Description and Use
X-Bar R	Two-part chart monitoring process accuracy and precision, e.g., patient waiting time and food temperature
p	Chart tracking acceptable or unacceptable process results as a percentage, e.g., percentage medication errors
N p	Unique p chart tracking acceptable or unacceptable process results, e.g., number of medication errors
c	Chart depicting an area of opportunity with occurrence held constant, e.g., number of reported accidents per day
u	Chart depicting an area of opportunity without holding each occurrence, e.g., number of misdiagnoses per DRG

ical example, while limiting focus on only those multidisciplinary tools and techniques required to support effective digital transformation of fundamental healthcare processes.

PROCESS CAPABILITY ANALYSIS

A process capability analysis is used to determine whether a process is capable of meeting an established specification as "controlled" by current natural variation. Being in control is not enough. An "in control" process can produce a bad product. True process improvement results from balancing repeatability and consistency with the capability of meeting patient or customer requirements. This approach objectively measures the degree to which a process is or is not capable of meeting those requirements. Capability indices graphically portray this situation by showing a distribution of process results or outcomes in relation to patient or customer specifications. Statistical control limits reflect current state process. A control chart is developed from a run chart modified to show average performance with process variation. Variance is expressed in standard deviations (i.e., square root of variance above and below mean performance over time).

> A square root of variation is a standard deviation (∂) and is calculated as the cumulative distance of values from a process's *arithmetic* mean, *not* its geometric mean.

SCATTER DIAGRAMS

This tool is used to examine relationships between two variables plotted as data pairs. A scattergram is used to test for *possible* cause and effect relationships by displaying patterns or possible relationships among data.

Although not proving that one variable causes another, a scattergram and an associated correlation coefficient demonstrate that a relationship exists and express the relationship's relative strength. When used in conjunction with a correlation coefficient, a scattergram describes and quantifies relationship strength between variables without expressing or demonstrating proof of any causal relationship (a scattergram is *not* a tool to be used to demonstrate a definitive cause and effect association). This technique is correctly used for continuous variables rather than discrete data.

Scattergrams are plotted for each data pair. Figure 2.11 is an example of a classic scatter diagram showing the number of billing errors compared with the number of overtime hours worked.

Each plotted point reflects a data pair of variables in a clustered pattern, with the "direction and tightness" of the cluster pattern expressing a type and relative strength of the relationship between each variable in each pair. As in this example,

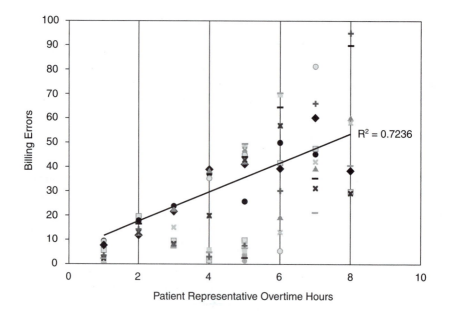

FIGURE 2.11   Scatter diagram (scattergram).

a straight line means that every time one variable changes the other would change by the same amount in the same direction, showing a stronger correlation between these variables.

After collecting 50 to 100 paired samples of paired data, horizontal and vertical axes can be drawn using commercial spreadsheet software to support development. A scattergram and associated correlation coefficient can be displayed and analyzed. A variable suspected as a possible "cause" is drawn horizontally and a possible "effect" variable is usually vertical. The resulting patterns and analysis are summarized as a graphic of all plotted pairs.

Figure 2.11 is an example of a scattergram produced from data pairs with a positive correlation of 0.72, implying that a possibly strong relationship exists between patient representative overtime hours (x-axis) and billing errors (y-axis). The degree to which an increase in x corresponds with a comparable increase in y is expressed as the correlation coefficient. A correlation coefficient indexed at exactly 1.00 is relatively rare.

Other possible types of correlation include the following:

- A negative correlation depends on the degree to which an increase in x corresponds with a decrease in y. A negative relationship is as important as a positive relationship.
- There is no correlation when the correlation approaches zero.
- A straight line correlation, as in Figure 2.11, is very common but is the only relationship that may be encountered. Nonlinear correlations require the use of additional statistical tools that are beyond the scope of this book.

HISTOGRAMS

This tool is used to analyze data by summarizing and presenting data as a frequency distribution in tabular form and graphically as a bar graph. Graphic formats of this type display either raw or aggregate data that are otherwise difficult to interpret in tabular form.

> Histograms are "intermediate tools" to assess data distribution (e.g., centering, spread, and shape).

- *Show* relative frequency of occurrence for a specified time period (e.g., hour, shift day, week, etc.)

- *Use* historical data to find patterns or to use a baseline measure of past performance
- *Reveal* centering, skewing variations, and the shape of underlying data distributions
- *Provide* useful information to assess current or predict future process capability and performance

Commercially available spreadsheet software includes functions to facilitate data collection, aggregation and analysis as a tabular frequency distribution, and display in a classic histogram format. Initial histogram interpretation includes analysis of data distribution centering or skewing and variation or spread. This analysis answers questions about the data, for example,

- Is the data distribution normal (bell shaped), bimodal (twin peaks), or multimodal (three or more peaks)?
- Is the process center running too high or too low relative to patient expectations, analytical specifications, or outcomes?
- Is the process too variable (i.e., within requirements)?
- Does the process demonstrate consistent performance?

Figure 2.12 is an example of a classic histogram as a specialized bar graph presentation of the same data set shown in Figure 2.11 as a scattergram.

TEAM DYNAMICS FACILITATION TECHNIQUES

Remaining tools and techniques in this chapter are less quantitative and more qualitative in nature. Each tool capitalizes on and uses these facilitation techniques to create ideas by harnessing the power of team dynamics and dialogue. This facilitation focuses team members on problem identification, analysis, and solution development.

These tools are used during and after initial brainstorming sessions or other group dynamics techniques from previous analyses (e.g., NGTs, cause and effect analysis, force field analyses, etc.). Some experts consider these techniques alterative or specialized forms of structured brainstorming.

Figure 2.13 shows a conceptual application of these group dynamics using a real-world example drawn from the design and development of the National Health Information Network (NHIN). This set of problem identification and solution development techniques is especially useful as each team member gains an understanding of potential issues that identify driving forces, priorities, and desired outcomes. These tools and techniques facilitate systematic identification, analyses, and classification and prioritization of potential influential cause and effect

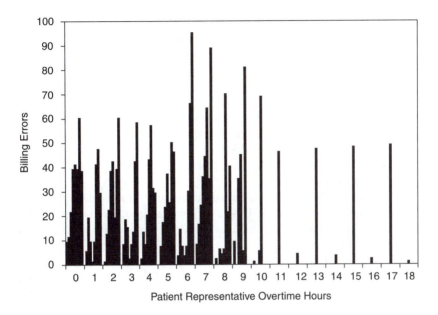

FIGURE 2.12   Histogram distribution of patient representative billing errors by overtime hours.

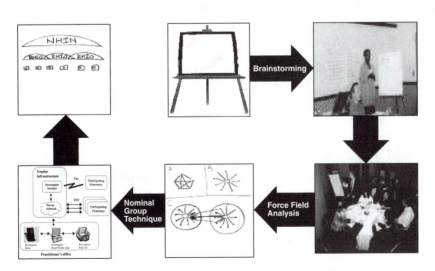

FIGURE 2.13   Using group dynamics tools to design an NHIN.

relationships that exist among and between critical issues. These key drivers or outcomes must then be incorporated as core components of a credible solution. These tools

- *Encourage* team members to think in multiple dimensions rather than only linear directions.
- *Enable* participants to explore cause and effect relationships among and between issues that may be controversial.
- *Require* a deeper exploration of key issues to naturally emerge rather than just superficial discussions of issues, potentially forced by dominant or powerful team members.
- *Identify* basic assumptions and underlying reasons for systematic disagreement among team members. This is an important process to ensure that a final solution inclusively incorporates key aspects from varying perspectives of each team member.
- *Facilitate* team identification of root cause(s), agreement, and focus on problem articulation and analysis even if credible empirical data do not yet exist.

These tools encourage additional discussion as may be required to ensure that input is valid and clearly understood by all team members. Groups use these tools to gain a comprehensive knowledge of subjects under discussion by considering whether resulting cause, priority, sequencing, and effect patterns ensure that their proposed solutions are more likely or less likely to be credible.

BRAINSTORMING

Brainstorming is used to initiate creative thinking by team members, operations analysts, systems analysts, and management engineers. Brainstorming sessions begin as both a team leader and a recorder are selected and the brainstorming topic is clearly and precisely stated.

> The objective of a brainstorming session is to generate as many ideas as quickly as possible without any consideration of each idea's quality, value, or merit.

Brainstorming is either structured or unstructured:

- Structured brainstorming requires every team member to contribute an idea in rotation or pass until the next round. This technique encourages even shy team members to participate but enables all present to contribute.

- Unstructured brainstorming permits contribution of spontaneous ideas as expressed by team members in any sequence. This technique creates a more relaxed atmosphere but risks domination by more vocal members.

The following guidelines are useful to maximize a brainstorming session:

- As ideas are generated, the recorder documents each idea so it is visible to all members. A common form of recording ideas is to print them on flip charts in large handwriting and then display multiple sheets taped to walls of meeting room.
- As everyone agrees on an issue or idea, it is recorded on the flip chart in words of each speaker without interpretation.

Brainstorming occurs in distinct phases: creation, refinement, and assessment. The creation phase is started by the team leader's review of appropriate rules, for example, individual ideas are posted in sequence, one at a time, without discussion or criticism. This phase continues until all ideas are exhausted. Team members may pass without expression of a new idea. Individual ideas frequently build on others, with this phase continuing until all ideas are exhausted. During refinement and assessment phases ideas are reviewed by all team members to ensure that everyone understands each idea without further discussion or criticism. This tentative idea list is reviewed during assessment discussion. This final phase eliminates duplication or issues that are not on topic. A structured series of votes should reduce the team's consensus list of ideas as much as possible.

CONTINGENCY DIAGRAMMING

This tool is used to refocus team analysis when members are grid-locked, when some or all present are hostile, or when a very controversial issue is being confronted for further analysis. Contingency diagramming contributes "group dynamics" to quickly find and resolve persistent problems with practical solutions. At times, individuals and groups may focus first on negative aspects of an issue, especially when confronted with a difficult problem or analytic resistance.

A contingency diagram uses reverse logic to generate promising solutions. This approach builds on brainstorming to identify as many ways as possible that a problem could get worse or persist. As a team works through this process, it gains systematic insight to solve the problem. An action plan is then quickly and easily prepared to prevent this problem from recurring.

Figure 2.14 illustrates an example of how this technique could be used to plan more effective team meetings. A flip chart is created in advance of a team meeting. This tool should be sketched as in Figure 2.14 with only the problem to be

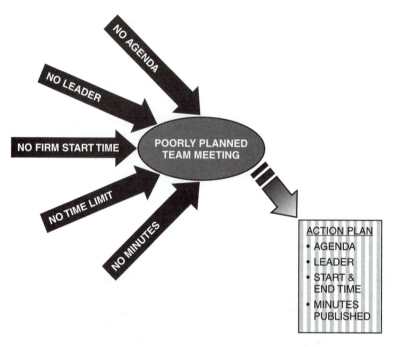

FIGURE 2.14   Example of contingency diagramming.

addressed in the oval. Using this technique a team's leader should initiate a structured brainstorming session to identify causes that would make this situation worse.

Effective use of a contingency diagram includes these key steps:

- *Ask* each group member to offer actions, permitting passing if a member does not express an idea.
- *Document* actions on "arrows" left of the oval.
- *Do not tolerate* any criticism, question, or praise of others' ideas during a brainstorming session. All present should refrain from comment, listen carefully, and courteously build on each other's ideas. Any input is acceptable, even silly, strange, or similar ideas. Great solutions frequently evolve as variations of other ideas.
- *Continue* until ideas are exhausted, recognizing that quantity of ideas rather than quality is the objective.
- *Clarify* ideas by team discussion while identifying actions that could prevent the problem from continuing by working through each *opposite* action.
- *Develop* an action plan to document corrective actions.

WHY TECHNIQUE

This simple tool is an effective approach to problem-solving that drills down through multiple but less obvious or unacknowledged cause levels. The why technique is used to identify a potential and preventable root cause of a recurring problem by simply asking why a problem occurs. The question of why the problem occurred is persistently continued until a root cause is targeted for further analysis and resolution. This technique is especially effective in potentially "confrontational" group settings.

Execution is simply repeatedly exploring cause levels through as many iterations as are required:

- *Focus* on a problem.
- *Ask* "Why did this problem occur?" to uncover a first-level cause.
- Repeat asking "Why did this problem occur?" for each cause to uncover a next layer of cause(s).
- *Strive* to uncover multiple causes at each level as each cause level is explored as a likely chain of events.
- *Continue* to repeatedly ask "Why?" until a root cause is identified for further analysis and resolution. If cause levels are exhausted without identifying a root cause, another technique is recommended for additional analytical focus.

The why technique is useful for both problem identification and analysis, as is the more graphic fishbone diagram.

NOMINAL GROUP TECHNIQUE

This group dynamics tool is frequently used to make decisions. A working definition of consensus is introduced and acknowledged by all present as "a solution that everyone can live with and no one is prepared to die for."

> Nominal group techniques are useful when a team must develop a consensus to identify priorities or to define a sequence of actions in rank order.

NGT fixes sequential relationships or priorities among and between topics, actions, or items. NGT is a common complement of previous brainstorming sessions. This "ranking approach" enables decision-makers to quickly come to a consensus on the relative importance of issues, problems, or solutions. This technique builds team commitment to a decision using equal participation and an agreed on process that aggregates individual rankings into a team's priorities. Each team member ranks issues without pressure by others.

By using this approach all team members are on an equal footing to clarify team consensus or lack thereof. This process complements brainstorming, especially with decisions involving sensitive topics. Causes of disagreement can be identified and addressed during this process and between multiple iterations of ranking.

Application of an NGT technique includes these elements:

- Topics or issues to be ranked or sequenced are written on a flip chart as the team eliminates duplicates and/or clarifies meanings.
- With the team's permission and guidance a final list of topics is identified with letters, not numbers, so that team members do not get confused by the numerical ranking process that follows.
- Each team member records these corresponding letters on a piece of paper and rank orders each topic with a numeric value, which may include zero if no value is associated with a topic. Conceptually, each member has one vote per item, but any member may choose to assign all their votes to a single or a limited number of items to be ranked.
- All team member rankings are then combined for each item to reflect each item's team ranking.
- Multiple ranking cycles may be necessary, especially when only a few choices must be selected or ranked from a large number of items.
- A consensus selection or rank is achieved when the team choice is clear.

FORCE FIELD ANALYSIS

When used after brainstorming, contingency diagrams, the why technique, or NGTs this approach clearly identifies barriers to process improvement recommendations. Force field analysis requires a team to acknowledge driving and restraining forces and then support the development of effective countermeasures. Force field analysis enables a team to develop a deeper understanding of organizational politics and existing culture. These considerations are critical when implementation strategies are being developed.

"Driving forces" are likely to support a proposed situation requiring behavior change, whereas "restraining forces" are likely to impede and present barriers to desired change. Without a desire for change, opposing or restraining forces may appear to be too strong and are likely to hinder any implementation initiative. By using this tool, dynamic team dialogue can creatively build on existing driving forces to counter negative perceptions that threaten the status quo. Figure 2.15 is an example of using force field analysis to build a justification for substantial capital investment for IT infrastructure and systems implementation.

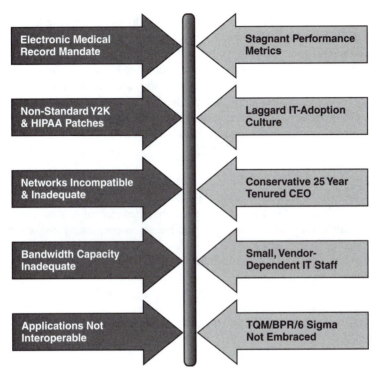

FIGURE 2.15 Information system investment justification.

Desired change requires that driving forces be stronger than restraining forces. Otherwise, change will not happen until countermeasures are tactically incorporated into implementation strategy. Desired change will only occur when driving forces are more powerful than restraining barriers to change. Effective development of this desired disequilibrium requires force field analysis to

- *Encourage* team members to think cohesively about all aspects of a desired change
- *Stimulate* creative thinking and collaboration on relative priorities of driving and restraining forces
- *Expedite* consensus building when used with other tools (e.g., NGTs, contingency diagramming, and why techniques)
- *Provide* a starting point for action

Encouraging effective change requires strengthening driving forces or reducing restraining forces. Resistance rather than desired improvement occurs when unintended consequences reinforce negative forces. Effective strategies and operational tactics must be developed and introduced to diminish or eliminate restraining forces. Teams are more likely to be successful when they identify and understand potential negative impacts before implementation. Having done so by using force field analysis enables teams to be deliberate and proactively plan actions and countermeasures rather than be forced to react if not anticipated.

SUMMARY

This chapter introduced data collection topics, analytic techniques, and team dynamics tools. When used in various combinations, these techniques generate active team collaboration that leads to effective decision-making by team consensus.

Fundamental concepts and content included

- Brainstorming
- Flowcharting and imagineering
- Force field analysis
- Ishikawa diagramming
- NGTs
- Pareto analysis
- Run and control charts

CHAPTER QUESTIONS

These questions reinforce student understanding, learning, and retention while stimulating class discussion:

1. Identify key symbols used for imagineering, and explain differences between process, horizontal and deployment flowcharts.
2. Define Pareto Analysis and discuss why this tool is both a problem identification and an analytic tool.
3. Explain the differences between a cause and effect, Ishikawa and fish bone diagram with examples.
4. In the context of statistical process control, how are common and special causes different?
5. What is process variation?
6. How is process variation related to process capability and customer expectations?

7. Explain how a traditional bell curve, a run chart, a control chart, and 1, 2 and 3 standard deviations are related.

8. What is meant by the terms "in-control" process and "out-of-control" process? Describe how they are different.

9. How is a scatter diagram constructed and what is its relationship to a positive and negative correlation co-efficient?

10. Identify three common group dynamics tools and explain how each technique is used.

11. Describe a situation when a team leader may use a contingency diagram.

ADDITIONAL RESOURCES

These references are recommended for additional reading and more comprehensive content beyond the scope of this book.

Barry, R., Murcko, A., Brubaker, C. (2002). The Six Sigma Book for Healthcare. Chicago: Health Administration Press.

Bassard, M., Ritter, D. (1994). The Memory Jogger: A Pocket Guide of Tools for Continuous Improvement and Effective Planning. Salem, NH: Goal/QPC.

Coile, Jr., R. (2002). New Century Healthcare Strategies for Providers, Purchasers, and Plans. Chicago: Health Administration Press.

Coile, Jr., R. (2002). The Paperless Hospital: Healthcare in a Digital Age. Chicago: Health Administration Press.

Dale, N., Lewis, J. (2004). Computer Science Illuminated. Sudbury, MA: Jones and Bartlett Publishers.

Deming, W. E. (1986). Out of Crisis. Boston, MA: MIT Press.

Goldsmith, J. (2003). Digital Medicine Implications for Healthcare Leaders. Chicago: Health Administration Press.

Griffith, J., White, K. (2002). The Well-Managed Healthcare Organization. Chicago: Health Administration Press.

Harrell, C., Bateman, R., Gogg, T., Mott, J. (1996). System Improvement Using Simulation. Orem, UT: Promodel Corporation.

Herzlinger, R. (1997). Market-Driven Health Care: Who Wins, Who Loses in the Transformation of America's Largest Service Industry. Reading, MA: Perseus Books.

Labovitz, G. (1997). The Power of Alignment. Billerica, MA: Organizational Dynamics.

Larson, J. (2001). Management Engineering. Chicago: Healthcare Information and Management Systems Society.

Longest, Jr., B., Rakich, J., Darr, K. (2004). Managing Health Services Organizations and Systems. Baltimore, MD: Health Professions Press.

MacInnes, R. (2002). The Lean Enterprise Memory Jogger: Create Value and Eliminate Waste Throughout Your Company. Salem, NH: Goal/QPC.

Martin, P., Tate, K. (1997). Project Management Memory Jogger: A Pocket Guide for Project Teams. Salem, NH: Goal/QPC.

Nelson, R. (1999). Tele-health: changing healthcare in the twenty-first century. Journal of Health Information Management, 13(4), p. 71–77.

Newell, L. (2000). Beyond Year 2000: Innovative solutions for the evolving healthcare information management environment. Journal of Health Information Management, 14(1).

NHII status. Retrieved June 29, 2007 from http://www.hhs.gov/go/healthit/

Null, L., Lobur, J. (2006). The Essentials of Computer Organization and Architecture. Sudbury, MA: Jones and Bartlett Publishers.

Seidel, L., Gorsky, R., Lewis, J. (1995). Applied Quantitative Methods for Health Services Management. Baltimore, MD: Health Professions Press.

Seymour, D. (2006). Futurescan Healthcare Trends and Implications, 2006–2011. Chicago: Health Administration Press.

Tufte, E. (1990). Visual Explanations. Cheshire, CT: Graphics Press.

Tufte, E. (1997). Envisioning Information. Cheshire, CT: Graphics Press.

Tufte, E. (1997). The Visual Display of Information. Cheshire, CT: Graphics Press.

Veney, J., Kaluzny, A. (1998). Evaluation and Decision Making for Health Services. Chicago: Health Administration Press.

Wan, T. (1995). Analysis and Evaluation of Health Care Systems: An Integrated Approach to Managerial Decision Making. Baltimore, MD: Health Professions Press.

CHAPTER 3

Information Technology: Components, Functions, and Features

This chapter introduces IT and focuses on these key concepts:

- IT capabilities, functions, and features
- Fundamentals of essential IT components
- IT memory, processing, and systems architecture
- Strategic transformation of digital functions using IT

Mastery of these concepts, tools, and techniques within these dimensions determines IT literacy of prospective IT professions:

- *Understanding* what a computer is as well as having a fundamental understanding of related technology terminology about systems, applications, functions, and capabilities
- *Demonstrating* a fundamental level of technical competency (performing and teaching others basic system operations that are necessary to complete assigned tasks)
- *Realizing* that significant organizational transformation occurs with an introduction or modification of IT
- *Acknowledging* systems, applications, processes, functions, and tasks performed require adoption of and adaptation to these changes with necessary encouragement of users to master new requirements

- *Acquiring* an awareness that appropriate IT application and utilization of IT in current and future healthcare delivery processes fundamentally impacts on the quality of human life
- *Understanding* that significant change occurs throughout, among, and between personnel and organizational and social structures when "disruptive technologies" are introduced
- *Appreciating* that these changes must be efficiently engineered to provide value, improve patient satisfaction, and increase organizational effectiveness

COMPUTER USE AND USER REQUIREMENTS

Widespread evidence of pervasive computer use is readily apparent in virtually all healthcare delivery organizations. For example, in hospital settings, admissions departments process information about incoming patients. Using computer terminals or personal computer networks, hospital representatives enter and/or update information about each patient (patient's name and other demographic information, insurance information, and a reason to be admitted to the hospital). This information is stored in the Hospital's Information System (HIS) to be retrieved as needed.

Group practices or health maintenance organizations electronically submit insurance claims for each patient's bill by using computer systems specifically designed for their practice or business. Medical secretaries and administrative assistants schedule appointments, transcribe medical reports, or use office computer systems for medical practice accounting. As the pace of digital transformation quickens in patient care delivery processes, exciting opportunities exist in these provider organizations and in other businesses providing products and services related to healthcare delivery.

Workers entering this workforce must be prepared to demonstrate an operational understanding of computer systems of all types. For example, medical transcriptionists operate word processors integrated with voice recognition software to prepare and edit documentation of care delivery dictated by clinicians. Nursing staff monitor patients' vital signs using wireless Personal Digital Assistants (PDAs), smart cellular telephones, or bedside computer terminals. Radiology technologists use advanced imaging technology to capture, analyze, and communicate information gain without invasive diagnostic and therapeutic patient procedures. Large research institutions employ many professionals with a variety of skills who are making new discoveries and advancing patient care options.

Healthcare team members work together, researching and delivering solutions to life-threatening problems in specialties such as neurosurgery, endocrinology, and cardiology. Computerized technologies of all types are used to facilitate patient specimen and data analyses and to rapidly produce information to support research activity of these teams. By decreasing time devoted to necessary but increasingly burdensome documentation and other administrative tasks, physicians are devoting more time to patients by practicing medicine with computer assistance equipped with more user-friendly technology. Federal mandates require digital creation, processing and transmission of insurance claims, and automated posting of paid claims to each patient's account.

Medical claims companies need qualified computer-literate workers with specialized medical training to analyze patient claims and documentation necessary to process and adjudicate medical insurance claims. Nurses are frequently employed to review medical records, collecting data archived for future utilization analyses. Specialized support services augment healthcare professionals (e.g., companies developing, producing, and distributing pharmaceuticals or other specialized equipment, such as hospital beds and wheelchairs). These businesses employ administrative and sales staff to market and distribute products. More intensive use of ITs of all types increases productivity and reduces cost. Specialized professionals need computer-literate support staff with combined medical backgrounds and IT training.

IT functions include acquiring, processing, and storing enormous amounts of information. As technologies have become ubiquitous, IT is increasingly commonplace in hospitals, clinics, laboratories, imaging centers, research facilities, and physicians' offices. Unfortunately, significant technology investment has not been and is not well integrated or interoperable. Current healthcare processes do not effectively support patient-centered, efficient, quality-driven, and affordable healthcare delivery.

PATIENTS DESERVE MORE, NOT JUST MORE TECHNOLOGY

Despite per capita expenditures that are consistently the highest in the world, America's health status is currently unacceptable, reflective of inefficient and ineffective care delivery systems and processes. Figure 3.1 is a bar graph showing that America has the highest healthcare expenditures as a percent of gross national product among developed nations. Figure 3.2 is a bar graph that highlights America's healthcare expenditures as the highest per capita among developed nations. Figure 3.3 is a scatter diagram comparing male life expectancy to annual per capita health expenditures. America is in the lower right quadrant, reflecting significantly higher expenditures and lower life expectancy outcomes (America spends the most per capita for health care and experiences the lowest male life expectancy among these developed countries). Life expectancy is but one of a number of health status indicators that are internationally accepted benchmarks used to demonstrate regional, state, or national healthcare delivery effectiveness.

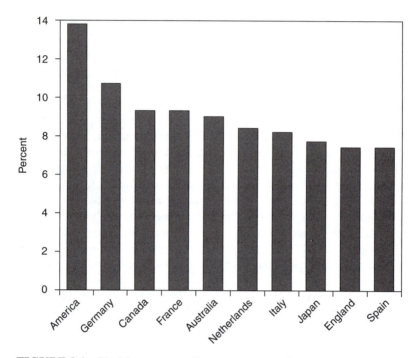

FIGURE 3.1   Healthcare expenditures as gross national product percent.

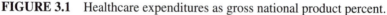

Current IT applications in America's healthcare provider organizations reflect more than 50 years of fragmented and collectively disjointed initiatives to reduce tedious routine tasks and improve efficiencies within individual departments. As a nation, America's healthcare delivery providers have not yet realized technology's virtually infinite potential to improve care delivery effectiveness. Based solely on this conclusion, radical redefinition is needed to integrate our fragmented processes into seamless patient-centric care delivery designs.

Without fundamental digital transformation of provider processes, the inefficient and expensive efforts to eliminate or further limit disease processes will continue to fall far short of otherwise unlimited potential. We have experienced profound scientific and clinical achievements that computers have enabled. Unfortunately, cumbersome and needless complexity also evolved from originally sound design that was simple, elegant, and effective. Frequently, these application installations were underfunded and forced by tight project deadlines. Such constraints

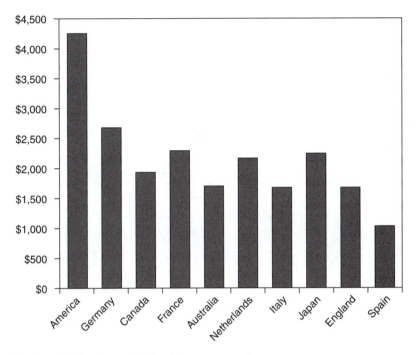

FIGURE 3.2   Per capita healthcare expenditures.

limited work process analysis and reengineering which would otherwise have resulted in efficient interfaces, seamless integration, and interoperability among key systems throughout most provider organizations.

To proficiently participate on any project team, aspiring IT professionals need to understand fundamental software and hardware functions, input and interface requirements, and output specifications. Through collaboration, team members gain a required appreciation of how a proposed solution will influence workflow effectiveness, efficiency, staffing requirements and timeliness, cost, and functions and feature trade-offs. IT professionals must be able to analyze, interpret, and present relevant operations research. These analyses should necessarily involve user, clinician, and patient interactions with each module of any system application. Benchmarking techniques are critical and applicable to proficiently evaluate technical hardware and software performance as well as user efficiency and overall care delivery process effectiveness.

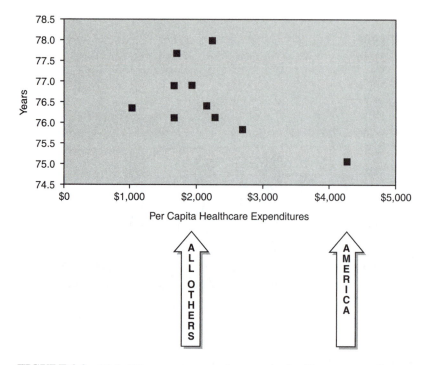

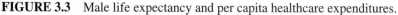

FIGURE 3.3   Male life expectancy and per capita healthcare expenditures.

SYSTEM FUNDAMENTALS AND COMPUTER APPLICATIONS

These reflections illustrate the need to gain an essential understanding and appreciation of how any computer works. Such learning begins with a fundamental definition of a computer: an electronic device capable of facilitating data input and performing manipulation, storage, calculation, comparison, communication, transformation, formatting, reporting, and presentation.

> An electronic device capable of facilitating data input and performing manipulation, storage, calculation, comparison, communication, transformation, formatting, reporting, and presentation.

Computers and computer systems are classified in different ways for different purposes, including size, type, function, and feature. Traditionally, size and processing capabilities were predominant characteristics of supercomputers, mainframe computers, minicomputers, microcomputers (i.e., desktop, laptop, PDAs, and, more recently, smart telephones). Technology trends reflect accelerated development of faster, more powerful multiprocessors with more dense and greater memory capacity, and smaller size that consume less power and generate less heat.

Supercomputers are very fast frequently networked systems capable of processing extraordinarily complex applications in healthcare research, robotics, national defense, weather forecasting, and artificial intelligence.

Mainframe computers are large systems capable of processing massive volumes of data. Initially, these computers were platforms for many legacy Hospital Information Systems (HIS). Originally, these computers supported administrative and financial applications in large hospitals (e.g., patient registration, scheduling, and claims processing), and, later, clinical applications. Mainframe computers have been characterized as those with faster processing speeds than either micro- or minicomputers. They also had much greater storage capacity, although more recent advances have diminished these distinctions. Costs of mainframes vary widely depending on their processing speeds and storage capacity. Historically, most providers used in-house mainframes for HIS and vender hosting of shared systems. These shared systems were configured with on-site minicomputers linked to mainframe systems supporting financial and clinical application in large remote data centers that operated for hundreds of provider organizations.

Minicomputers are characterized by larger storage capacity, faster processing speeds than microcomputers, but with a smaller size than mainframe systems. Many departmental systems were and still use minicomputers with fast processing speeds interfaced to clinical instrumentation and other networked technology. Many mid-sized and small hospitals and large physician group practices use minicomputers for core applications. Some legacy systems are hybrid minicomputer and networked solutions.

Microcomputers (i.e., personal computers [PCs]) are in widespread use in virtually every healthcare organization and venue and are quite capable of functions previously relegated to legacy mainframe and mini-systems. They are ubiquitous, versatile, flexible, and quite commonplace. They may be network servers and clinical instrument interfaces and are common replacements for legacy video-terminals. Based on Moore's Law as explained in detail by Dale, Null, et al., additional resources increased processing power, faster speeds, and more storage options are growing at an extraordinary pace with phenomenal numbers of transistors packed on each microchip. Computing power, speed, and storage capacity that was only available with early mainframe systems are now common in laptops, notebooks, PDAs, and smart telephones. As IT research continues to develop faster, smaller, and less expensive options, this pace of innovation accelerates with multiprocessor devices, nonsilicon processors, photon and biologic-based computing with optical circuits replacing electron-based computing.

> Information systems are groups of interoperable components, applications, and associated technologies working together to complete a set of specified tasks.

Although it is sometimes difficult to distinguish between hardware issues and software issues, computer design algorithms (mathematic, logical, or algebraic expressions) are software programs written in a "high-level" fourth-generation or higher computer language. As such, a computer program is a structured set of sequenced algorithms, in which a "nested" algorithm produces an algorithm and another algorithm that runs that algorithm and so forth until instructions are executed as a series of 1's and 0's at the machine level. An algorithm at the machine level operates as an electronic device. Because of this hierarchal structure, algorithms are best understood as "nested" instructions to perform ever more fundamental tasks that might otherwise have been manually executed by a user.

Thus computers are implementations of algorithms that execute other algorithms, and this chain of algorithms leads to this principle of equivalence:

Anything that can be done with software can also be done with hardware, and anything that can be done with hardware can also be done with software. Even more fundamentally, anything done by a computer's hardware and software can also be done by a human or a group of humans if time, precision, and accuracy are not limiting factors.

Although this principle does not explicitly address the speed with which these equivalent tasks are completed, hardware implementations are almost always faster and software executions are usually faster than manual processing.

More fundamentally, data input must be represented in language that a computer can understand and process. Each keystroke must be translated into machine language before processing, with information processed as a binary digit, or a bit. When an electrical charge is present, a bit has a value of 1. When no electrical impulse is present, a bit is 0. Bits are grouped to make a byte, representing a single machine language character.

Data are collected, processed, and stored to meet process, function, application, or program requirements. Data processed by computer systems are controlled by programs directing this digital transformation into useful information for analytic action. Information results from data or facts that are collected and processed. Data are input to a computer's system memory component via input devices and processed in a system's central processing unit. Information output is used, produced, or processed further through other computer programs or applications after data processing completion.

A data processing cycle results as information is stored in secondary storage for immediate action or for later use. Output may become input for further processing operations. Identical data may be collected and processed by various other programs, applications, or computers to produce different information depending on organizational requirements.

Facts, or data, are organized in a variety of ways to provide useful information. For example, when a patient receives a procedure as ordered by a surgeon, supplies are consumed. Procedures and supply items are charged and will appear as a charge with a clinical procedure terminology (CPT) code on this patient's final bill. Based on this charging process for supplies consumed, a purchase order is generated via a materials management application. This is then transformed into a SKU-coded purchase order that is transmitted to a preferred supply vendor's system, which replenishes inventory for this item. This process is a materials management life cycle.

This example details how identical data or facts reflect different informational needs within and between provider departments and external organizations. Each digital module involved in processing these discrete data is defined as functions performed within a data processing cycle (order entry, surgical scheduling, billing, accounts receivable, and materials management).

A basic understanding of fundamental computer hardware components and key functions of *any* computing device (mainframes, minicomputers, desktops, laptops, handheld PDAs, and smart cellular telephones) is required working knowledge for all IT professionals. Any computing device consists of three essential components.

The first component is a *processor*, which interprets and executes programs by supervising and managing all operations, communicating through circuitry that oversees execution of commands to begin, perform arithmetic or logical operations, and terminate each operation or task upon execution:

- Arithmetic operations are mathematical calculations of addition, subtraction, multiplication, and division.
- Logical operations involve three essential comparisons based on decisions when values are greater than, less than, or equal to each other.

The second component is *memory*, which stores programs and data:

- Primary memory stores data and program instructions, without performing any logical operations. Different terms may identify primary memory, such as primary storage, memory, main, or internal memory.

- Memory can be **random access memory (RAM)** or **read-only memory (ROM)**. RAM is **volatile memory**, and stored data are lost if electrical power is interrupted.
- **Cache memory** is buffer storage of frequently used data blocks that are closest to a Central Processing Unit (CPU).
- Cache is volatile memory and may be **virtual memory**. Virtual memory is a physical extension of main memory that is designated on another storage device to "enlarge" cache beyond physical limitations to concurrently run more processes.
- Shared memory residing with multiple processors may be accessed as a single entity, enabling inexpensive "supercomputing capability."
- ROM is not volatile and includes basic instructions to start or "boot" computer operations. ROM can be **firmware** with hardware and software characteristics.

Memory is measured in bytes, kilobytes, megabytes, or gigabytes. Data and program instructions are stored in primary storage and moved as necessary for processing. Computer memory is hierarchically organized (i.e., larger, slower, and less costly as well as smaller, faster, but more costly memory). Most computers include some combination of cache, main memory, and secondary memory (e.g., disk and/or tape drives, optical disks, digital video disks), as successive hierarchical layers.

The third component is a *mechanism* that transfers data to and from an external environment:

- *Hardware* is any physical component used to process data (e.g., CPU, memory, keyboard, mouse, display, buses, printers, displays). Hardware includes devices for input, output, processing, and storage of data. Examples of peripheral devices are monitors, disk drives, compact disks or digital video recorders, keyboards, scanners, and printers.
- *Software* is a set of programmed instructions directing system hardware components to complete data processing tasks.
  - Systems software controls system operations by directing, commanding, scheduling, and confirming data processing functions. Systems software includes operating systems and specialized programs such as utilities, programs, or translators.
  - Applications software includes programs performing specific data processing functions, usually for end-user functions.

These three key elements are required in all systems to perform data processing and transform data into useful information.

More advanced memory and processor relationships include

- Data flow computers that enable data to drive computation
- Neural networks that learn to execute computations via arrays of processing elements which continue until computations are completed
- Biologic, optical, and quantum computers developing computing concepts (see Chapter 15)

A processing cycle includes all data collection, through input, and processing task to various types of output, as well as all associated manual and computerized functions and tasks.

A clock is a vital system component that keeps all system processing synchronized. Clocks simultaneously send electrical pulses to key components, ensuring that data will be where expected and instructions executed as expected. These pulsations are frequencies emitted each second measured in cycles per second, or hertz. When system clocks generate millions of pulses per second, they operate in the gigahertz range. As of this writing, processors in typical desktop and laptop computers are operating in the gigahertz range, generating billions of pulses per second.

Frequency ratings are benchmarks of microprocessor speed and are determinants of overall system performance. Similarly, networking speed reflects time devoted to file-sharing or communicating with peripheral devices (e.g., scanners or printers).

A simple analogy is a class with each student functioning as a computer with these three computer components: a brain as a processor, class notes as memory, and pen and paper representing transfer mechanisms. Instructor-to-student, student-to-instructor, and student-to-student interactions during a class discussion are analogous to a transaction transported on a network. When an instructor poses a question, this question is recognized and documented (stored) by each student and discussed among the class. When concluded with a correct response to the instructor's question, this process is representative of a "data processing" cycle.

FUNDAMENTAL SYSTEM TERMINOLOGY AND OPERATIONS

A basic understanding of measurement terminology, although specific to computer applications, is fundamental knowledge required of all transformationalists because automated applications function in an analytic context of process efficiency, process capability, and workflow. The National Institute of Standards and Technology approved standard names and symbols to differentiate binary and decimal prefixes early in the IT evolution. Table 3.1 highlights key prefixes and symbols.

For example, a small word processing file may be 50 Kb in size, a graphic image, a 4-Mb object, a flash or hard disk drive 2 Gb in size, or the distance

TABLE 3.1   IT Prefixes and Symbols

Prefix	Symbol	Power of 10*		Prefix	Symbol	Power of 10*	
Kilo	K	Thousand	*[3]	Milli	m	Thousandth	−[3]†
Mega	M	Million	[6]	Milli	μ	Millionth	−[6]
Giga	G	Billion	[9]	Milli	n	Billionth	−[9]
Tera	T	Trillion	[12]	Milli	p	Trillionth	−[12]
Peta	P	Quadrillion	[15]	Milli	f	Quadrillionth	−[15]
Exa	E	Quintillion	[18]	Milli	a	Quintillionth	−[18]
Zetta	Z	Sextillion	[21]	Milli	z	Sextillionth	−[21]
Yotta	Y	Septillion	[24]	Yocto	y	Septillionth	−[24]

*1,000
†0.001

between transistors on a microchip 48 nm apart. Processing speed or microchip cycle times are expressed in terms of fractions of a second (e.g., thousandths, millionths, billionths, or trillionths as fractional prefixes on the right side of Table 3.1). Exponents are reciprocals of these prefixes depicted on the left side of Table 3.1. As a simple example, if an operation requires a microsecond to complete, then a million operations occur within a second.

An understanding of these fundamental computer operations is essential. IT professionals must understand and demonstrate multidisciplinary competency to effectively facilitate team leadership and be able to communicate these concepts to application users and senior executives.

Effective digital transformation of healthcare delivery processes depends on IT professionals to lead team discussion and collaborate about system capabilities, strengths, and limitations. Mastering basic computer applications and dependent issues require given appropriate attention, deliberation, and decision-making for results to produce effective process redesign and achieve project objectives.

Healthcare IT professionals must meet these challenges of digital transformation of care delivery with demonstrated computer literacy and competency. Virtually all healthcare diagnostic, therapeutic, or treatment protocols, applications, policies, and procedures are computerized and increasingly dependent on information systems at an ever accelerating pace. All IT professionals must be computer literate, be able to define what a computer is, know how to operate a computer to perform professional and administrative tasks, and appreciate the social and ethical impacts that IT has on individuals and society.

In summary, a data processing cycle refers to each stage of data transformation of information. The input stage, often referred to as data entry, occurs when data are first introduced into a computer system. Processing refers to data manipulation that occurs in the CPU to produce output as data or, more importantly, as information. Storage is retention of data or information in either a volatile or permanent form.

Processing may occur in different time frames. *Off-line processing* occurs at intervals, and information is not always current or readily available in real time. Online systems are real-time systems in which processing occurs immediately so that data input are current and virtually occur simultaneously.

Data can be processed in many ways to produce desired output. Information system operations produce information by processing data, including calculations, input, output, query, classifications, sorting, updating, summarizing, storage, and retrieval. Online processing is real-time interactive or transaction data processing without any delay, as processing occurs immediately upon the availability of input and output transactions. Processing of input transactions and processes typically occur in transaction input sequence order. Frequent feedback to users with "front-end edits" produces more accurate data input because input is validated online in real-time communication with a CPU.

Online processing occurs through a direct connection between terminals and CPU. Off-line processing systems do not provide direct communication with a CPU. Online systems are connected to a CPU via "online" terminals for data input or for receiving output. These online terminals may be a personal computer (PC), a video display terminal, a cathode ray tube (CRT), a "client" or "dumb terminal," or another such device.

Batch processing is an off-line application or system that stores data for processing at periodic intervals. For example, a payroll system using batch processing may collect information available on hours worked for all employees in advance of processing paychecks and associated reports at the end of a pay period. Batch processing is useful for certain applications, such as payroll or billing systems, when information does not need to be available on a real-time basis. Batch processing is relatively inexpensive and an efficient method for processing large data sets.

Data processing, aggregation, and organization reflect data transformation into meaningful information using basic data processing operations. Brief descriptions of these fundamental data processing operations follow:

- *Calculation* transforms data into information through mathematical calculations. For example, monthly patient billing statement totals can be added together to provide an accurate annual assessment of patient revenues.
- *Input* requires data entry via a variety of hardware devices into a system's CPU arithmetic–logic unit where processing operations are executed.

Regardless of the input device used, data input must occur before other data processing operations can occur. Many input operations are by data entry.

- *Output* generates information by transforming organized data into a useable form (a letter or a monthly revenue report). Output may be digital, hard copy, or both that can be printed or written to a compact disk or other more permanent media. A digital or "soft copy" is information displayed on a computer monitor and is not a permanent copy because it is only temporally retained in volatile memory. Output operations are performed by a variety of hardware devices.

- *Query* or *inquiry* is a request for information performed by keying a command or a key word associated with information to be accessed.

- *Classification* is grouping data as being meaningful and useful. Classifying simply organizes data into categories (e.g., alphabetical or male and female designations). Numerical codes often represent classifications (e.g., a numerical classification system might be CPT codes, which are numerical codes representing medical procedures).

- *Sorting* is a specialized classification operation that arranges data in a sequence or specified order. Common sorts include alphabetical or numerical listings, first to last, high to low, small to large, and so on.

- *Update* is a change in stored data to reflect more current conditions (updating, editing, or revising involves adding, deleting, or modifying existing information). For example, making an update to a patient's previous address in a HIS.

- *Indexing* creates a file-based key field while leaving original data intact by creating a pointer field within an indexed file to establish, maintain record sequence, and reestablish an original position of a record in an original file. Fields include both a record number and a pointer in each original file. An end of file indicator means that there are no more records. For example, to create an indexed file patient zip codes are in ascending order fields to be sorted, and after sorting record numbers and pointer fields change position. An original file is maintained in proper sequence through the pointer field.

- *Summary reporting* includes counting and totaling fields within files to provide counts, subtotals, and totals.

- *Exception or ad-hoc reporting* selects records within a file that reflect a unique characteristic to be studied. Patient care information systems are designed so that authorized users may specify and execute these reports as needed with a "report writer."

- *Detail reporting* includes listings of every record within a file, including category subtotals and totals. System documentation typically outlines a report's content and format (line spacing, tab settings, and any unusual features). Fields to be calculated are usually specified along with calculation instructions.

Database constructs or database architectures reflect structure, format, and organization of data storage within each database of an HIS application:

- *Relational* databases use existing relationships among and between individual records by identifying *key* record field(s).
- *Hierarchical* relationships are established among records as a "tree structure" (a top level record is identified as a "parent" record and is related to lower level "child" records).
- *Networked* databases use network structures to relate records when database fields reside physically or virtually on different processors within an integrated delivery system (IDS) network.

As IT evolved from relatively simple general-purpose calculating devices into increasingly sophisticated applications, a standardized hierarchy of different levels of software and functions became necessary to understand and explain system architecture at different levels. Each level in this hierarchy defines "semantic gaps" between high-level programming applications and physical attributes of computer components (microchip circuits, buses, gates, and wires). These levels are numbered from 0 to 6, where 0 represents machine-level operations and executable programs with which IT professionals must be familiar. Table 3.2 summarizes these seven layers.

HEPIS (HEALTHCARE E-PATIENT INFORMATION SYSTEM)

The remaining sections of this chapter describe system modules, applications, and functions in a narrative summary. Some combination or frequently updated versions of these applications operate in healthcare provider organizations. Table 3.3 highlights these capabilities at an application level, and Figure 3.4 depicts common interactions and interfaces of these modules as a high-level schematic. In the remaining chapter narrative more detailed descriptions of each application are given, including typical functions and features. In the context of these descriptions, as well as elsewhere throughout this book, a comprehensive legacy HIS alludes to various characteristics, functions, and features of the Healthcare E-Patient Information System (HEPIS).

A digitally transformed information system implies this minimal set of IT capabilities, functions, and features. An IT configuration of these or comparable functions and features is necessary to provide effective, patient-centric, and state-of-the-art healthcare information management technology to a digital transformation of any provider organization. Capabilities, applications functions, and features in this comprehensive but not all-inclusive example describe a typical provider information system currently operational in hundreds of

TABLE 3.2 Systems Operations Hierarchy

Level	Content	Functions
6	User level consists of applications and is the level of functions and features with which most everyone is familiar.	User run programs (e.g., word processors, spreadsheets, databases, graphics packages, games, internet browsers, etc.). Only level visible to users.
5	High-level languages (e.g., C, C++, Cobol, Fortran, M, Pascal, etc.) that are either compiled or interpreted to a machine language. Compiled languages are translated into assembly language, then assembled machine code.	Programmer knowledge about data types and instructions available and how they are implemented.
4	Assembly language level is compiled from higher level languages (i.e., translated to machine language).	Each assembly language is translated to one machine language instruction consisting of 1s and 0s.
3	System software (i.e., operating system responsible for protecting memory, multiprogramming processes, and comparable functions).	DOS, Leopard, Linux, Unix, Vista, Windows.
2	Instruction Set Architecture (i.e., machine language) recognized by particular system architecture.	Programs in native machine language executed directly by hard-wired components without compilers or interpreters.
1	CPU control unit verifies that instructions are decoded and executed properly so that data are where and when instructed.	CPU interprets each machine instruction, one instruction at a time, and executes each action as instructed.
0	Digital logic within system physical components.	Fundamental hardwired mathematical logic (e.g., chips, gates, and buses).

provider organizations throughout the nation. This level of system functions and features is required to support effective digital transformation of care delivery processes throughout a typical healthcare provider organization. Specific functions and features have been available as turnkey solutions from numerous commercial vendors for many years. These specific applications, functions, and features are presented to explain system capabilities in sufficient descriptive detail of operational or proposed functions and features (required functional

TABLE 3.3   HEPSIS Applications

Accounts Payable	Master Patient Index
ADT Logistics	Materials Management
Adverse Drug and Allergy Interaction Tracking	Medical Record Abstracting/Coding/Imaging
Benefits Administration	Nursing: Progress Notes, Lists, Staffing, Vital Signs
Budgeting, Financial, and Operations Modeling	Nutrition, Dietetics, and Food Service
Cardiology Information Management	Order Communication
Case Mix Analysis, Management/Modeling	Results Reporting
Chart Efficiency Tracking/Locator	Quality Outcomes Management
Clinical Data Repository	Patient Registration, Scheduling, Accounting
Clinical Documentation/Decision Support	
Clinical Reminders, Discharge Tracking	Personnel/Payroll Processing/Premium Billing
Computerized Patient Record	Pharmacy Information, Management Applications
Cost Accounting and Resource Management	
CPOE	PACS
Decision Support: Operations/Planning	Point-of-Care/Bedside Terminals
Dictation/Transcription	Productivity/Resource Management
Electronic Medication Administration	Radiology Information Management Applications
Eligibility Verification/Claims Management	Resource Scheduling
Emergency Information Management	Social Services/Case Management
Executive Information/Dashboard	Simulation: Operations Research/ Forecasting
Human Resource Information Management	Surgery Scheduling/Information Management
Intensive/Critical Care Patient Monitoring	
Laboratory Information Applications	Time and Attendance
Laboratory Instrumentation Data Collection	Voice Recognition/Transcription/ Documentation
Managed Care Contract Management	
Market Research, Demographic Demand Modeling	

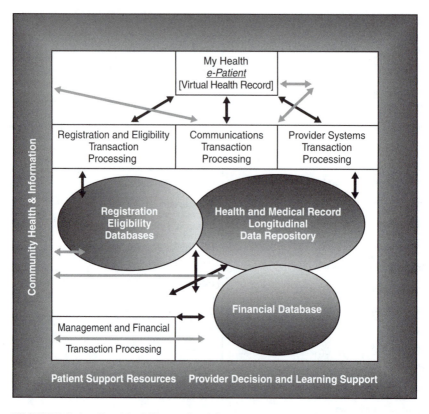

FIGURE 3.4   Graphical illustration of the Healthcare E-Patient Information System (HEPIS).

content for a request for proposal [RFP] to replace an outdated legacy system). Although obviously very rich in technical capabilities, this system specification, including these applications as described, is available to any qualified healthcare provider organization at nominal cost.

HEPIS supports a true longitudinal healthcare record, including data from both in-network and out-of network sources. HEPIS supports research and population analyses and facilitates patient access to data and sharing of information to improve data quality, consistency, and integrity in a securely networked environment throughout multiple provider entities within an IDS.

HEPIS serves as an operational clinical repository (e.g., a cohesive portfolio of clinical information), incorporating both in-network and out-of network provider data that resides on one or more independent platforms to be used by clinicians and other personnel to facilitate longitudinal patient-centric care. Data in HEPIS is organized in a format supporting timely and effective care delivery in virtually any venue, regardless of patient or provider location or a patient's clinical information. These HEPIS applications, modules, functions, and features transparently support patient-centric care delivery processes using industry-standard interfaces within an interoperable integrated network environment.

HEPIS's "e-Health" application functions support a variety of customer-friendly patient-centric capabilities, such as prescription refills, appointment scheduling, and online forms completion, as well as patient and provider access to health records, online health assessment tools, and high-quality real-time health information. These capabilities are representative of digitally transformed care delivery.

HEPIS provides significant additional benefits beyond seamless automated support of care delivery. It also provides information to support demographic research and population analyses, facilitating patient access to data and information sharing. HEPIS enhances IDS capabilities by improving data quality and security and minimizing mundane administrative costs.

Admission, Discharge, Transfer, and Registration

This comprehensive array of functions and features is dedicated to administrative functions for patient admission, discharge, transfer, and registration. Admission, discharge, transfer (ADT) modules provide functions to be used throughout each patient's acute inpatient, long-term care, and/or outpatient stay. Registration, enrollment, and eligibility applications are designed as a single IDS-wide data system and demographic database that supports comprehensive registration and eligibility verification, thereby ensuring information consistently and accessibly in all other applications in the HEPIS network.

Automated Medical Information Exchange

This module facilitates electronic interchange of patient information among and between providers and facilities and retains timely, accurate, and comprehensive audit trails of information exchange. This module includes several key components, such as provider- and facility-specific administrative options, applications, and components that enable efficient daily reporting and maintenance.

Authorization/Subscription

HEPIS utilities support identification and tracking of transactions by authorized personnel to perform various actions on clinical documents (e.g., signing, cosigning, and enhancing text and image definition requirements).

Care Management

This HEPIS application offers care providers inquiry capability to view pertinent information about multiple patients on a single screen. With this function, users can view multiple patients requiring attention:

- *Clinician dashboard* is a table of patients for whom clinicians have unacknowledged results or event notifications (admissions, discharges, or unscheduled clinic visits, unsigned documents, or uncompleted tasks).
- *Nurse dashboard* provides a similar list of patients for whom nurses have unacknowledged results, unviewed events, uncompleted tasks or text orders, unverified orders, or recent vital signs.
- *Query tools* enable authorized users to create reports based on most current patient data via defined user-created custom reports.
- *Sign list* enables authorized users to approve multiple actions for multiple patients. For example, clinicians can sign a discharge summary for one patient and notes for another. Predefined reports include abnormal results, consultation status, incomplete orders, and recently scheduled activities.

Case Registries

Registries contain key demographic and clinical indices for patients identified by provider with specified diseases and/or disorders based on primary, secondary, or tertiary International Classification of Disease, Version 9 (ICD-9) and Version 10 (ICD-10) coded diseases and disorders or CPT coded procedures. These registries extract from HEPIS databases (e.g., pharmacy and laboratory) and provide key clinical information. Data are used to track and optimize clinical care of patients receiving care by various providers in multiple venues.

Clinical Monitoring System

This module enables users to capture and monitor patient data as required by various quality management initiatives. Typically, patient data are automatically captured from an existing database and edited to track specific events. Statistical data are maintained for each patient scanned, determining the number of patients meeting monitoring criteria, by selected data trending for user-specified time frames (hourly, daily, weekly, monthly).

Clinical Procedures

This application uses HL7 messaging to pass final patient results between commercial clinical information systems and displayed patients' test results. Discrete report data are stored in HEPIS databases to share data and images with other HEPIS modules (consult/request tracking, text integration utilities, patient care encounters, and HEPIS imaging packages). Clinicians may document findings and complete final procedure reports generated by medical devices. These key functions enable clinicians to enter, review, and continuously update order-related information for any patient. Patient allergies or adverse reactions to medications are recorded, as well as requests for and tracking consultations status, progress notes, diagnoses, treatments, and discharge summaries for each patient.

Integration with other HEPIS applications facilitates accurate and timely record-keeping and compliance with clinical guidelines and patient medical record requirements. Authorized personnel maintain comprehensive patient records enabling clinicians, managers, and quality assurance staff to review and analyze data to directly support clinical decision-making. Adverse reaction tracking is a common and consistent data structure to detect and monitor adverse reaction data. Options expedite data entry and real-time validation and references used by both HEPIS and external systems to report adverse drug reaction data to the U.S. Food and Drug Administration (FDA).

Clinical Reminders

Clinicians can provide and receive appropriate and timely patient treatment reminders to assist clinical decision-making and educate providers about appropriate care options. Electronic clinical reminders improve documentation and follow-up, enabling authorized providers to view test or evaluation results and track and document care as ordered and delivered. This capability reduces duplicate documenting activities, assists in targeting patients with particular diagnoses and procedures using site-defined criteria, and assists in compliance with clinical care guidelines. Consultation and request tracking enables clinicians to efficiently order and track real-time status of consultations and procedures from other providers or services within each clinical setting in any in-network venue.

Health Summary

Health summaries are clinically oriented structured reports that extract and abstract data from HEPIS databases and use a standard format to display information and report information. Health summaries are printed or displayed for individual patients or groups of patients. Displayed data include user-defined health-related information such as demographic data, allergies, active medical problems, and test results. Data and summary information are integrated with clinical HEPIS applications and modules.

Health summary functions export components to authorized staff who can remotely view patient data. Clinical reminders are integrated with health summary functions to inform providers with timely information about each patient's health maintenance schedules. Clinical providers collaborate with authorized technical staff coordinators to configure customized schedules based on local and national clinical guidelines. Health summary components such as past progress notes are available to display new interdisciplinary progress notes and relevant entries.

Home Care

This is an optional module designed with secure remote entry and verification of patient-related data from home care providers delivering care in patient homes or other in-network facilities. This module's design uses a relational database structure, incorporating wireless security to ensure data integrity and access accountability.

Imaging, Radiology, and Nuclear Medicine Applications

These function-rich applications provide seamless real-time imaging by automating diagnostic and therapeutic services. Examples of key features include patient registration for examinations, order entry and service requests, image processing and interpretation, automatic request tracking, result recording and reporting, and online report verification, display, and printing of recurring ad-hoc statistics and management reports.

- Remote order entry functions support chain order fulfillment production.
- HEPIS applications and associated databases integrate clinical, administrative, and business processes (e.g., contracting and acquisition management, order fulfillment, distribution management, finance, and equipment life cycle management).
- Extensive order tracking, serialized device registration, and service history are available.
- Scheduling automates appointment and scheduling processes, including procedure setup and maintenance, enrollment, scheduling, and resources. Messages are displayed as an appointment is scheduled (e.g., notification that an appointment is an overbooking, conflicts reporting, etc.).
- Imaging applications enhance and expedite medical decision-making by delivering integrated multimedia patient information to each clinician's desktop. Imaging transmits high-quality image data for many specialties (cardiology, pulmonary, and gastrointestinal medicine, pathology, radiology, hematology, and nuclear medicine).
  Imaging processes textual reports as scanned documents and electrocardiograms. These HEPIS imaging capabilities are integrated and interoperable with other applications, providing a comprehensive electronic patient record

that is accessible to authorized clinicians any time and anywhere. Imaging improves patient care and enhances both quality and timeliness of clinician communication, daily conferences, educational seminars, and patient rounds.

- Diagnostic imaging displays are used for enhanced digital film-less interpretation of radiology studies and for radiology workflow management. Imaging includes a variety of core components.

- Core infrastructure includes components used to capture, store, and display images captured from video cameras, digital cameras, document and color scanners, x-ray scanners, sonograms, and files created by commercial capture software. Images are directly acquired from Digital Imaging and Communications in Medicine (DICOM)–compliant devices such as computed tomography, magnetic resonance imaging, positron emission tomography, and single photon emission computed tomography and other additional digital radiology equipment. Captured images are accessible throughout all venues with a compliant graphic user interface on clinician desktops. Associated images are automatically accessed when viewing a procedure or examination report or progress note.

- DICOM text gateways provide patient and order information to medical devices (e.g., computed tomographs and digital radiography systems to expedite each examination performed). Data provided by these DICOM text gateways comply with all industry-wide DICOM modality work-list standards. These DICOM text gateways enable patient and communication of order information to any commercial picture archiving and communications system (PACS) within an IDS network as well as to out-of-network clinicians. DICOM image gateways securely receive images from external PACS systems or acquisition devices. Image gateways transfer images to DICOM-compliant storage devices for display, printing, or teleradiology purposes:

  - Enabling online availability of all information in an electronic patient record, including immediate availability of critical documents to authorized personnel (e.g., advance directives and informed consent forms) at any time in addition to handwritten papers, drawings, signed documents, and medical correspondence

  - Linking to and scanning of paper-based patient information to electronic patient records such that all patient information is expeditiously available and easily retrievable from a single source

  - Potential savings due to reduced medical records staffing requirements and filing costs as well as minimizing lost or misfiled medical chart information

  - Sustainable benefits include decreased retrieval and delivery functions, reduced volume of paper records, and rapid information accessibility for clinicians

Background processing manages image storage on network devices. An imaging database links images and electronic patient records, including magnetic storage via redundant array of independent disks and optical jukebox storage for archives.

Intake and Output

This application design stores patient intake and output information for each hospital stay or outpatient visit. This application is not service specific and is integrated with appropriate HEPIS modules.

Incident Reporting

This module supports organizational policies by compiling data on patient incidents and organizing data into defined categories for reporting and tracking at each provider facility level and for transmission to quality assurance databases for corporate office review and tracking.

Laboratory Applications

HEPIS' clinical laboratory applications provide laboratory data and formatted information to clinicians as required to support specimen collection; analyze, report, interpret, and evaluate clinical implications; and provide high-quality, efficient, cost-effective timely patient care. These modules enable clinical, technical, and administrative personnel to effectively manage increasing automation and robotics driven by heavier workload to be completed faster with fewer resources while continuing to enhance laboratory processes and reporting. Modules support clinical laboratory, chemistry, hematology, immunology, and microbiology. Instrument interfaces are industry standard for virtually all routine high-volume procedures. Web-enabled links are available via secure networks to expedite logistics to and reporting from reference laboratories at any location.

HEPIS' Surgical/Anatomic Pathology Laboratory module provides automated record-keeping and reporting for surgical pathology and anatomic pathology, histology, cytology, electron microscopy, and autopsy. These functions enable staff to improve quality management, increase productivity, use and provide comprehensive research and reporting capabilities, and facilitate workload management and statistical reporting.

Blood banking functions use data tied primarily to a donor, a patient, or a unit of blood/blood component. Information about a blood donation or a donation attempt includes demographics and potential risk history of each blood donor. Similarly, accurate and timely information about each unit of blood or blood component in inventory requires effective real-time unit identification and location. Transfusion and testing information involves patient sampling and associated blood or blood component administration.

Nutrition and Food Service

Nutrition and food service applications integrate automation of clinical nutrition, food management, and management reporting functions. HEPIS supports activities such as nutrition screening, nutrition assessment, diet order entry, tube feeding and supplemental feeding orders, patient preferences, diet pattern calculations, nutrient analysis of meals, consultant reporting, and quality of care tracking. Food management functions include total automation of food acquisition, production activities, service, distribution, inventory, cost management, recipe expansion, menu and recipe nutrient analysis, meal and diet pattern development and implementation, diet card and tray ticket printing, and service quality tracking. Meals served, cost per meal, tube feeding cost, supplemental feeding cost, staffing, encounter data, information query and summary capabilities, and annual management reporting are also reported.

Patient Representative Applications

Patient-centric and patient representative design ensures that providers and facilities respond to unique patient needs while tracking and trending patient compliments and complaints. This module measures the facility's types of complaints as they relate to effective customer service standards. These functions collect and categorize complaints and compliments with components that identify opportunities to meet and exceed each patient's expectations. Issue codes provide tracking capabilities for complaints and trends of specific complaints. Customer service standards can be tailored to include unique issue and reliability studies. These studies drive initiatives to improve patient perception tracking and extract specific data for each provider, department, nursing unit, outpatient clinic, product line, or service.

From registration or admission eligibility determination through discharge by online real-time data transmission to optimize reimbursement for care with comprehensive DRG and resource utilization group (RUG) functions and features, these functions support collection of patient information, including demographics, employment, insurance, medical history and associated data. Other modules (e.g., laboratory, pharmacy, radiology, and nursing) use information gathered through various ADT options. These features optimize operational efficiency while limiting unauthorized user access to specified sensitive patient records. A patient sensitivity function permits a level of security to be assigned to certain records within HEPIS databases to control unauthorized user access. Efficient and expeditious retrieval of patient records incorporates identification of potential duplicate patient entries.

Accurate real-time collection, maintenance, and output of patient data enhance a health care facility's capability to provide quality patient care. Key capabilities include patient registration, bed management, tracking of inpatient movements, inpatient care groupings (DRGs), and outpatient groupings.

Patient Inquiry and Eligibility

HIPAA Title II compliant telecommunications networks can respond to authorized requests to obtain patient eligibility data for individuals or groups. These networks process the payer requests from provider computers to payer networks and validate patient eligibility and claim information to determine patient insurance coverage, thus expediting claim adjudication upon patient discharge. Claims data for high-volume payers (e.g., Medicare, Blue Cross, Medicaid) are transmitted in virtual real-time directly to a payer's network. Lower volume payer eligibility and claim processing transmissions are routed by electronic batch through commercial clearinghouses for claims processing and to apply payer-specific coding and formatting. An online suspense file stores requests for later transmission and records payer responses, thereby logging relevant activity. By using this robust capability to obtain patient eligibility information quickly, accurately, and efficiently, clinicians are authorized to act expeditiously to provide urgent and emergent patient care and to recall and store diagnosis, medical treatment, and related therapy. Returning data from payers and clearinghouses are loaded directly into HEPIS databases and queried by authorized personnel throughout the IDS. Various screens in key modules display data in a returning payer message and information currently on file for comparison.

Patient Record Tracking

This module enables authorized staff to maintain medical record control and expeditious record availability to users throughout the IDS. A vast array range of facility, provider, and authorized individual definable parameters support custom tailoring to meet specific needs in any setting. This module is fully integrated and interoperable with other HEPIS applications (e.g., radiology and pharmacy). Automated filing functions support all clinical and relevant administrative activities. Representative features of this module include requisitioning activities for individual records within and among IDS facilities, including creation of new records, charge-out/check-in of records, inactivation and reactivation and deletion of records, printing of bar code labels, transfer of records to other in-network and out-of-network facilities, recharging records to other borrowers, and flagging missing records.

Patient Identification Card

This application identifies patients with a color photograph and encrypted patient demographics to initiate care and service processes in all in-network care venues within the IDS. A print option provides labels with a patient's key identifying information on bar-coded labels affixed to medical record forms. This color photograph uses nationally standardized patient image capture software (PICS) on a CCOW-enabled workstation.

Population Health

This application is an optional module that computerizes, tracks, and aggregates data for all venues. An automated assessment capability captures and reports various longitudinal aspects of care provided (e.g., care efficiency, care outcomes, and care quality). These reports

- *Enable* clinicians to determine differences in disease frequency between individuals and among selected cohorts in a population
- *Provide* information to support clinical guideline development
- *Support* health screening guidelines for patients and populations
- *Collect* and *report* workload data, preventive screening, outcome measurement, and provider profiling data

Problem List

Problem list capabilities include documentation and tracking of patient problems. These functions provide clinicians with current and historical views of healthcare problems across clinical specialties for each identified problem traceable throughout HEPIS for treatment, test results, and outcomes.

Resident Assessment/Minimum Data Set

This long-term care module provides a standardized, comprehensive, accurate, and reproducible patient assessment tool as a fundamental baseline as a resident's plan of care is developed. This module streamlines data collection processes with acute care, rehabilitation, and skilled nursing facilities as required by the CMS using a nationally standardized minimum data set (MDS). Versions are defined by CMS to receive Medicare or Medicaid reimbursement using standard HL7 messaging.

In addition, this module provides a structure that meets the JCAHO long-term care accreditation standards and provides opportunities and data comparison capabilities for resident outcomes. This module incorporates the nationally standardized HL7 gateway interfacing to import and export data triggered by specific MDS responses in multidisciplinary care plans. The MDS generates version-specific RUGs and a variety of quality indicator reports.

Pharmacy Applications

Pharmacy functions are seamlessly integrated throughout the IDS and are complemented with extensive comprehensive HEPIS applications. This module's key functions are as follows:

- Automatic pharmacy replenishment/nursing unit stock tracks drug distribution and inventory management throughout each facility, venue, and IDS services. Key capabilities include inventory management for clinical care locations and drug crash carts.
- Medication administration capabilities include real-time point-of-care bar coding solutions that validate administration of unit dose and intravenous medications. This comprehensive automation and process control significantly increases more accurate and efficient administration documentation.
- Controlled substance management functions monitor and track receipt, inventory, and dispensing of all controlled substances by identity, using a list as a perpetual inventory of controlled substances. For example, when pharmacy personnel receive a controlled substance order, quantity-on-hand and receipt history is automatically updated.
- Authorized nursing staff order controlled substances via on-demand requests and receive these orders with secure delivery by pharmacy staff. Pharmacists dispense controlled substances using automated forms that complete each order request.
- Integrated medication management supports both intravenous and unit dose. These integrated functions provide a comprehensive record of medications used by patient and provider. Physician order entry enables authorized pharmacy staff to customize these functions and optimize productivity by facility, user, and medication.
- Intravenous medication management functions improve pharmacists and staff efficiency and accuracy with labels, manufacturing worksheets, and order updates by nursing unit lists.
- Unit dose medication management provides a standard computerized and, where appropriate, automated system for dispensing and managing inpatient medications. Timely, accurate, accessible, and up-to-date patient medica-

tion information is available to authorized personnel through each facility. Computer-generated administration worksheets enable nurses to dedicate more time to patient care.

- An IDS-wide formulary standardizes all local drug files, including adoption of updated drug nomenclatures and drug classifications, and links file updates to industry standards via data in the National Drug files approved by the FDA. Real-time access to information concerning dosage form, strength, unit, package size and type, manufacturer's trade name, and National Drug Code (NDC) information improve staff accuracy and timeliness of service.
- Outpatient pharmacy functions enhance management capabilities for outpatient medication regimens and manage and monitor workload and cost.

Surgery

This comprehensive set of applications is used by surgeons, surgical residents, anesthetists, operating room nurses, and other surgical staff. These HEPIS applications are integrated with other clinical modules supporting on-line real-time access to each patient's clinical record in surgical suites in the IDS.

Key functions including scheduling surgical cases and tracking inpatient and outpatient clinical data provide an integrated user-definable variety of reports. Nursing functions include intraoperative reports and automatic production of postoperative reports.

- Automated scheduling provides better operating room utilization and equitable distribution operative room schedule as well as ad-hoc, monthly, quarterly, and annual surgical reports. These capabilities reduce administrative overhead for clinicians, managers, and administrative support staff. Reporting capabilities include morbidity, mortality, and complication tracking.
- Risk assessment and performance tracking compare facility performance to national benchmarks for analyses of user-defined criteria such as observed-to-expected mortality, risk-adjusted outcomes, and morbidity ratios for all operations by specialty and subspecialty.
- Process simulation and model development is robust and dynamic, enabling management to monitor trends and to analyze and compare with national benchmarks.

Vitals Signs and Measurements

This nursing system application facilitates capture, retention, and reporting of key vital signs and various measurements associated with each patient's hospital stay or outpatient visit. Each patient's EMR includes these indexed statistics.

SUMMARY

This chapter included an overview of computers and their functions and features as well as information systems data structures and organizational hierarchy components and concepts. Computers were defined as electronic devices capable of rapidly and reliably processing and transforming data into information. Information systems are functional applications or units working together to perform data processing tasks. Systems are classified by size. Supercomputers are the largest, and mainframe computers are large computer systems capable of rapidly processing very large volumes of data. Minicomputers are smaller than mainframes but are capable of fast processing speeds and providing relatively large storage capacities. Microcomputers are smaller desktop systems, laptop computers, handheld computers, and smart telephones.

Data are defined as raw facts entered and stored in a system. When processing has been performed, output is information as a product. Data are represented in a form that computers understand. Digital computers process bits and bytes. Coding occurs during input and translates characters into machine language that CPUs process.

Fundamental concepts and content focused on

- Overview of IT capabilities, functions, and features
- Fundamentals of essential IT components
- IT memory, processing, and systems architecture
- Strategic transformation digital functions and IT

CHAPTER QUESTIONS

These questions reinforce student understanding, learning, and retention while stimulating class discussion:

1. Identify key characteristics of RAM, ROM, cache, and flash memory.
2. Explain differences between online and batch processing, especially strengths and shortcomings of each.
3. Define a computer and identify three key components and how they interact.
4. Explain Moore's Law and the Equivalence Principle as well as their relevance to the digital transformation of healthcare delivery.
5. Identify and briefly describe 10 of the 25 key applications of HEPIS.

ADDITIONAL RESOURCES

These references are recommended for additional reading and more comprehensive content beyond the scope of this book.

Coile, Jr., R. (2002). New Century Healthcare Strategies for Providers, Purchasers, and Plans. Chicago: Health Administration Press.

Coile, Jr., R. (2002). The Paperless Hospital Healthcare in a Digital Age. Chicago: Health Administration Press.

Dale, N., Lewis, J. (2004). Computer Science Illuminated. Sudbury, MA: Jones and Bartlett Publishers.

Goldsmith, J. (2003). Digital Medicine Implications for Healthcare Leaders. Chicago: Health Administration Press.

Null, L., Lobur, J. (2006). The Essentials of Computer Organization and Architecture. Sudbury, MA: Jones and Bartlett Publishers.

CHAPTER 4

Networking to Digitally Transform Healthcare Communication

This chapter introduces networking concepts, strategic communications infrastructure, and regulatory mandates. Essential network capabilities, components, and architectures are described in this chapter. Without imposing unnecessary burdens associated with fundamental yet complex technical discussions, these concepts focus on

- A multidisciplinary understanding of these sometimes technical concepts
- Networking definition and critical components
- Common topographies within and among healthcare providers
- Multidisciplinary applications to transform and integrate patient-centric digital communications
- HIPAA transactions, privacy and security mandates, implications, and requirements

NETWORKS

A network is a collection of computing devices connected to facilitate communication and sharing of resources.

Commonly shared tangible resources include servers, routers, modems, multiplexers, video-codecs, data storage devices, printers, scanners, facsimiles, and other multifunctional peripheral devices. Electronic mail, instant messaging, microwave, file-sharing, and Internet browsing all require communication across computer networks and represent common examples of tangible, intangible, or virtual resources.

Wireless network communications use radio waves or infrared signals without physical connections. Hard-wired connections commonly include twisted-pair wires, coaxial cables, or fiber-optic cables. A node or a host is a generic term used to describe any device connected on a network.

Bandwidth is a measure of information-carrying capacity of a network that is frequently associated with velocity or speed (transfer rate with which data are moved from one place to another on a network). Data are transferred as messages or "packets" along, among, and between network components connected in a variety of ways (network topology).

Message-passing efficiency is a key characteristic associated with network infrastructure that impacts process improvement and is commonly characterized by

- **Bandwidth:** carrying capacity that is maximized with data compression techniques
- **Message and transport latency:** time required for the first bit of a message to reach a destination and total time a message spends in a network
- **Overhead:** activities required to move a message from a sender to a receiver
- **Protocols:** well-defined rules that control data formatting and processing
- **Gateway:** node controlling communication between networks

Networks that are continually connected with networked components are connected to all other components are very expensive to build and difficult to manage, modify, and maintain. Network design is used to minimize network connections and distances that each message must travel between a sender and a receiver.

To improve information transferring efficiency over a shared communication link or line, messages are divided into a fixed-sized number of packets. Packets are individually sent over a most expedient network route to their designation, after which they are aggregated and reassembled into the original message.

Individual packets of each message travel different routes to a destination and are likely to arrive in a different sequence from that which was sent. Therefore each message is reassembled (i.e., reordered) and then combined to form the original message. This technique is referred to as packet switching.

COMMON TOPOLOGIES

Three topologies are commonly used in healthcare delivery networks. *Star configurations* use a central hub through which all messages must pass (Figure 4.1). While providing excellent connectivity, this central hub is a bottleneck. *Ring*

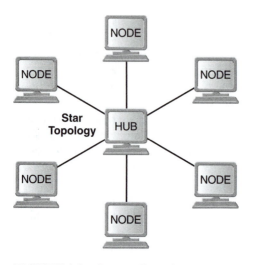

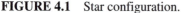

FIGURE 4.1   Star configuration.

configurations are a variant of linear arrays in which two ends are directly connected (Figure 4.2). *Bus configurations* are very common in local area networks (LANs) in which all nodes share a common line (Figure 4.3). The Ethernet is the standard for LANS.

More sophisticated and increasingly more complex configurations, including linear array configurations, permit any node to directly communicate with other nodes. These configurations enable all other communication through multiple entities:

- *Mesh networks* link each node to four (i.e., two-dimensional) or six (three-dimensional) nodes.
- *Tree networks* hierarchically arrange nodes as non-cyclic structures, creating multiple bottlenecks.

NETWORK CATEGORIES AND CONFIGURATIONS

Networks are also categorized, organized, managed, and controlled in various configurations:

- LANs are very common, most frequently using an Ethernet bus configuration topology (all nodes sharing a common line).

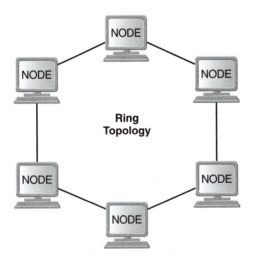

FIGURE 4.2   Ring configuration.

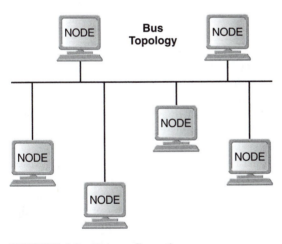

FIGURE 4.3   Bus configuration.

- Wide area networks (WANs) connect two or more local area networks, potentially over large geographic distances. WAN communication among and between smaller LAN networks use gateways to direct message communication.

- Metropolitan area networks (MANs) are required wireless network infrastructures deployed in large cities and surrounding suburbs.

  The Internet is a very large complex WAN spanning the globe, connecting many MANs and WANs with virtually infinite and redundant arrays of gateways, routes, and nodes. Providers and users of this vast array of networks have agreed to communicate with a common internet protocol (IP) to pass messages to and from senders and receivers to virtually any location worldwide and into space. No individual, organization, or single entity owns or entirely controls the Internet. The Internet backbone refers to a set of very-high-speed networks carrying Internet traffic. These networks are provided by large companies. Internet backbone networks operate at very fast data transfer rates, ranging from 1.5 megabits per second to more than 600 megabits per second. In some very specialized circumstances (very secure, secret, and highly classified military applications) data are transferred in gigabits or terabits per second via special optical cables and synchronized satellite links.
- Internet service providers (ISPs) are organizations that provide other organizations or individuals with Internet access. ISPs connect directly to the Internet backbone or frequently to larger ISPs with connections to the backbone. Internet service continuity is critical, requiring ISPs to provide redundant interoperable connection capability.

A variety of technologies provide Internet access, connection, and communication capability to residential and small business networks and stand-alone computers. Common techniques are sequentially faster with higher bandwidth and include telephone modems, digital subscriber lines (DSLs), satellites, or cable modems. Larger healthcare providers connect via dedicated T1 or T3 lines provided by local or regional telephone companies.

Local, regional, national, and international telephone system connections existed globally for voice communication long before Internet connections were necessary. As a result, the initial technique for network communication was a telephone modem. A **modem** is a *mod*ulator/*dem*odulator device that converts outgoing digital computer data into analog audio signals (modulation) for transfer over a telephone line and then converts incoming analog signals (demodulation) into digital computer data. One audio frequency is used to represent a binary 0 and another to represent a binary 1. Codecs perform a similar function for video images.

This approach was and remains relatively easy to implement because no telephone company effort or special expense is required. Because data are treated as if it were a voice conversation, no special translation is needed except at either end. However, only very low slow data transfer rates are available, usually 64 kilobits per second as limited to analog voice communication. This transfer rate became unacceptable for most Internet communications. In response, telephone companies began to offer faster DSL service. DSL became an increasingly popular approach within a limited distance from a telephone company's central office switch (i.e., a specially configured computer). As of this writing, the most common residential Internet connections are cable modems and satellite services with digital data transferred via existing cables or satellites used for television service.

HIPAA

The final section of this chapter is devoted to implications of significant regulatory mandates affecting network and communications security and privacy in healthcare delivery. HIPAA Title II, "Administrative Simplification," is the "accountability" portion of HIPAA.

HIPAA requires that providers and vendors support standardization for electronic submission of healthcare information with associated privacy and security safeguards. This federal regulation mandated dramatic changes to the use of technology that standardized transactions. These changes triggered increased concern about privacy of personal health information. As the federal government recognized HIPAA as an opportunity to encourage and facilitate electronic healthcare transactions, companion regulations defined standards for privacy and security of health information.

"Administrative Simplification" mandated new concepts and legal requirements for transmission, storage, use, and disclosure of health information. Because of the pervasive nature of these changes, substantial organizational and cultural changes were required for healthcare "covered entities." HIPAA compliance is required for covered entities (health plans, clearinghouses, and providers) transmitting health information in electronic form as a "covered transaction." A covered transaction is an electronic transmission of information between two parties to carry out financial or administrative activities related to health care.

Transaction standards define format, content, and consistency of healthcare-related electronic transactions and were expected to reduce inefficiencies in electronic information transmission. Implementation of this regulation has been viewed as industry-wide cost-savings opportunities to simplify and encourage electronic data transfer. These national standards are simplifying many processes associated with transactions. Table 4.1 summarizes the most common transactions used by hospitals, physician offices, and other covered entities.

These transaction standards are compliant with standard ASCI X12N formats used in other industries (e.g., banking and insurance). Parenthetical numbers reference these standard mnemonic formats.

Privacy standards regulate use and disclosure of protected health information (PHI) and still remain controversial, vague, complex, and the least understood

TABLE 4.1 HIPAA Transactions

• Claims (837)	• Referral Certification/Authorization (278)
• Payment/Remittance Advice (835)	• Health Plan Enrollment/De-enrollment (834)
• Eligibility (270/271)	• Health Plan Premium Payment (820)
• Claim Status (276/277)	

HIPAA regulations. Privacy standards apply to any electronic, paper, and oral communication of any individually identifiable health information transmitted or maintained in any form. Individually identifiable health information is any information relating to delivery of or payment for health care from which an individual may be identified.

Privacy standards impact organizational cultures and documentation related to privacy and confidentiality protections for patients. HIPAA privacy dictates detailed, specific, and comprehensive requirements that govern use of PHI consent forms, authorization forms, patient rights, privacy notices, business associate/ partner arrangements, and appointment of privacy officials. HIPAA training and tracking of training for a covered entities' workforce is required.

Security standards mandate safeguards for all health information pertaining to an individual that is electronically maintained or transmitted by a covered entity. The security and privacy standards are complementary because security policies, procedures, and technologies that mandate covered entities to keep PHI confidential. Security requirements include administrative safeguards, physical safeguards, and technical safeguards.

HIPAA SEVERITY MANDATES

These are selected policies and procedures that are required of each covered entity to be in compliance with HIPAA security mandates:

- Administrative requirements
- Physical safeguards
- Technical security services
- Physical safeguards
- Assigned security responsibility
- Media controls
- Physical access controls
- Policies and guidelines for workstation use and workstation location and for ongoing security awareness training

Preservation of PHI integrity is the primary focus of each security standard. These standards are intended to ensure that PHI cannot be altered, misused, or destroyed, either intentionally or accidentally, either during transmission through computer networks or at rest in any storage medium. Compliance with the HIPAA security standard requires appropriate technology and physical security measures (data backup, restricted system access through passwords, or encryption to maintain data availability).

SUMMARY

This chapter introduced terminology, tools, techniques, and concepts that explain networking configurations and communication operations and their applicability in healthcare provider organizations.

Fundamental concepts and content focused on

- Networking definition and critical components
- Multidisciplinary applications that transform and integrate patient-centric digital communications
- Implications of HIPAA transactions, privacy, and security
- Common topographies within and among healthcare provider organizations, as well as those necessary to support the community

CHAPTER QUESTIONS

These questions reinforce student learning, understanding, and retention while stimulating class discussion:

1. Define a network and describe three common topographies.
2. How are HIPAA privacy and security regulations related?
3. List and explain common HIPAA transaction standards.

ADDITIONAL RESOURCES

These references are recommended for additional reading and more comprehensive content beyond the scope of this book.

Dale, N., Lewis, J. (2004). Computer Science Illuminated. Sudbury, MA: Jones and Bartlett Publishers.

Griffith, J., White, K. (2002). The Well-Managed Healthcare Organization. Chicago: Health Administration Press.

Larson, J. (2001). Management Engineering. Chicago: Healthcare Information and Management Systems Society.

Longest, Jr., B., Rakich, J., Darr, K. (2004). Managing Health Services Organizations and Systems. Baltimore, MD: Health Professions Press.

Newell, L. (2000). Beyond year 2000: innovative solutions for the evolving healthcare information management environment. Journal of Health Information Management, 14(1), 1–24.

Null, L., Lobur, J. (2006). The Essentials of Computer Organization and Architecture. Sudbury, MA: Jones and Bartlett Publishers.

CHAPTER 5

Quality Management

This chapter focuses on these key concepts:

- Definitions of quality
- Quality Management (QM), process reengineering, and Six Sigma
- Quality pioneers
- Conformance and nonconformance costs of quality
- Benchmarking

Quality definitions vary, reflecting unique organizational cultures and objectives for patient care delivery. Like beauty, quality is in the "eye of the beholder." In this case the "beholder" is a patient with both real and perceived needs, wants, desires, and expectations.

In various organizations quality has been defined as

- Doing right things right, at the right time, every time
- Patient focus, total involvement, measurement, systematic support, and continuous improvement
- A blinding flash of the obvious

CHOOSING TOTAL QUALITY

Widespread use of public quality report cards and other competitive imperatives are demonstrating that hospitals providing poor care must rapidly improve and publicize implementation of corrective countermeasures to survive. Hospitals reporting superior care delivery must continue to improve to preserve their competitive edge, as other more typical hospitals are improving cost-effective quality care to avoid public perception as poor providers delivering high-cost low-quality care.

81

To become a superior provider of high-quality patient care, relationships must link Quality Management (QM) and productive providers, staffing, and effective and efficient processes. IT professionals must understand emerging technologies as key drivers of organizational change and lead these initiatives by using the theories, tools, and techniques presented in this book.

Virtually all basic QM tools are used in process design, process redesign, process improvement, business process engineering, and Six Sigma initiatives, as discussed in this and following chapters. Each process or application to be studied, its strategic criticality, defined project scope or perceived value, and available resources, sensitivity, time limits, and expected outcomes dictate the type and necessary rigor of process improvement that is most appropriate.

Figure 5.1 is a decision tree used to select an appropriate approach for each process improvement initiative in any venue for any provider organization. Figure 5.2 depicts expected outcomes to be anticipated from QM, business process reengineering (BPR), and Six Sigma initiatives. Each approach increases performance improvement to be achieved with varying degrees of rigor, application intensity, resource requirements, and IT applications, together with cultural change, time commitment, and financial investment. Figure 5.3 is an overview of foundational underpinnings as required steps in any approach to process improvement that can be sustainable over time.

LEADERS AND LEGENDS

QM uses quantitative and qualitative tools and techniques to systematically improve organizational performance on a continuous basis. Original concepts, techniques, tools, and analytics developed and refined by W. Edwards Deming and Joseph Juran have been applied with increasing intensity in service industries during the last 30 years. Key contributions by these men and other healthcare leaders influenced widespread adoption of these management philosophies and process transformation variants throughout health care. Compared with all other service industries, health care was late to embrace QM concepts and then only after mandated by the JCAHO.

This composite definition incorporates key elements found to describe QM's pervasive nature when effectively deployed in healthcare provider organizations:

> QM is a management philosophy and process improvement approach that focuses and commits managerial resources to a patient-centric, team-driven collaborative approach that strives to meet or exceed patient, internal and external customer expectations.

Effective application of any variant of this definition to achieving desirable outcomes in any healthcare provider organization requires that senior leaders,

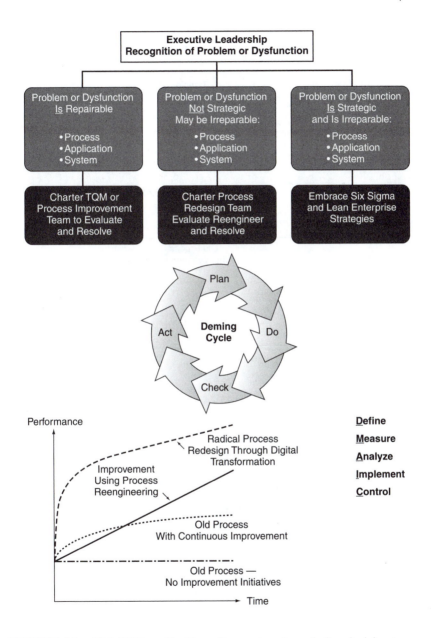

FIGURE 5.1   QM, BPR, or Six Sigma/lean enterprise solution decision tree.

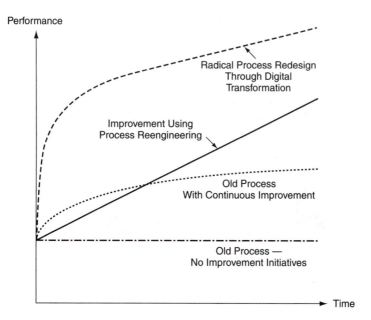

FIGURE 5.2   Anticipated outcomes of QM, BPR, or Six Sigma initiatives.

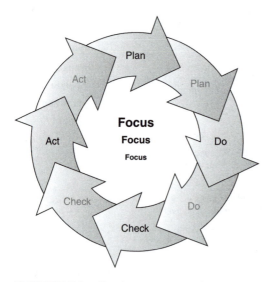

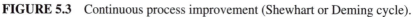

FIGURE 5.3   Continuous process improvement (Shewhart or Deming cycle).

mid-level managers, and "front line" supervisors visibly embrace a QM philosophy. Consistently "walking the talk" demonstrates a high level of commitment with leadership by example.

QM requires both structure and process (e.g., established and defined approaches and methods) based on continuous process improvement initiatives (i.e., application of *kaizen*, Japanese for continuous as opposed to breakthrough improvement). Patient-centric quality care must become a systemic focus to digitally transform processes, using these tools and techniques with systems, applications, functions, and features. Organization-wide emphasis must shift from inspection to prevention with everyone consistently striving to prevent defects before they occur. Staff training and ongoing retraining is critical to organizational improvement for each process so that errors or defects are eliminated and do not reoccur.

Fundamental philosophical perspectives and classic approaches pioneered by these QM legends are an appropriate beginning to understand and to achieve credible QM that can digitally transform provider organizations in patient-centric delivery systems. W. Edwards Deming believed that management's primary role is to coach employees. Education and training are staff investments to necessary reenergize staff, and avoid employee burnout, while articulating that management considers each staff member to be a valuable resource. Healthcare organizations must demonstrate a strong commitment to organizational transformation by investing in employees. Until this investment is openly demonstrated by senior leaders, employees will not embrace process level changes to effectively yield necessary digital transformation of healthcare processes.

DEMING'S STRATEGY AND PROCESS VARIATION

Senior management must focus on variability within existing processes to understand the scope and magnitude of required transformation in an organization. Deming's classic strategy builds on an organization-wide systemic understanding that *reducing process variation improves quality*. Process variation is of two types:

- Special variation caused by avoidable factors that cannot be ignored
- Common cause variation due to chance (i.e., inherent to an existing process) or to unavoidable and inevitable circumstances (e.g., mistakes, complaints, accidents)

Recognizing differences between stable and unstable systems is necessary to effectively manage an organization-wide digital transformation. A stable system is one whose performance is predictable or is said to be "in statistical control." Establishment and maintenance of stable system problems can only be addressed by management. Deming believed that continuous improvement enhances productivity through waste reduction and rework delays.

These concepts are commonly encountered throughout process improvement literature attributable to Deming's core beliefs:

- *Create* a constancy of purpose toward improved services while planning to become competitive, as is necessary to stay in business and provide jobs.
- *Adopt* a new philosophy reflecting a consumer, patient-centric, competitive environment in which currently acceptable delays, mistakes, defective materials, and defective workmanship are no longer tolerated.
- *Require* statistical evidence to demonstrate that built-in quality mass inspections are eliminated.
- *Eliminate* purchasing decisions that are based solely on price. Rather, depend on meaningful quality metrics to build loyal, long-term, and trusting relationships with a single supplier or "preferred partner" for each service or supply.
- *Increase* quality and productivity that systematically drive down costs by consistently improving systems, processes, and services, establishing and sustaining innovative techniques and processes through ongoing supervision and training.
- *Drive* out fear with training and teamwork, enabling staff to anticipate and resolve problems.
- *Eliminate* arbitrary numerical goals, work standards, and quotas by removing barriers and slogans.
- *Provide* process improvement tools and techniques to increase workforce productivity and develop a pervasive pride of workmanship.

Any credible patient-centric commitment to high-quality care delivery requires organization-wide participation that focuses these classic Deming concepts to

- *Demonstrate* management commitment, involvement, and leadership by providing quality improvement opportunities for all employees, physicians, and service providers
- *Identify* and *anticipate* future patient needs as well as those of internal and external customers
- *Delegate* responsibility and authority to improve processes to those actually doing the work
- *Create* multidisciplinary cross-functional work teams responsible for design, development, and improvement of policies, procedures, systems, applications, and processes
- *Commit* to measuring and monitoring patient care delivery quality by establishing process, results, and outcome measures and developing measures with patient and internal and external customer participation
- *Establish* and *monitor* key cost-of-quality indicators to continuously build, evaluate, and improve a quality infrastructure that parallels management structure

- *Manage* processes by linking quality to existing strategic planning, management, and performance systems, striving for excellence with recognition, reward, and celebration
- *View* all care delivery as process and make continuous improvements to better meet patient needs with benchmarking and innovation to achieve process improvement breakthroughs

COST OF QUALITY

Joseph M. Juran recognized nonquality costs, for example, reworking defective products and services, legal liability, and lost sales from previously dissatisfied patients or other customers who are purchasing competitors' products or services because of better quality. Juran, like Deming, pioneered QM as a trilogy of quality planning, control, and improvement over time.

Juran's experiences parallel the **Pareto principle** that at least 80% of quality defects are caused by management controllable factors. Caldwell, Juran, and others have demonstrated that quality components are attributable to strategic, controllable, or uncontrollable organizational defects, as depicted in Figure 5.4.

Juran viewed chronic waste as opportunities for improvement, stressing that deliberate action is required to seize opportunity. Quality improvement is a process beginning with identification of chronic quality problems. As identified, each need for change and improvement must be effectively communicated to others to build support for a necessary change throughout the organization.

Alternative solutions are next identified and analyzed, with each option analyzed to identify the recommended one that is expected to produce best results when implemented and sustained through continuous improvement. Ongoing control can only be sustained by continuous monitoring to ensure ongoing improvement.

Juran recognized that hands-on management and training are fundamental requirements to achieve and maintain excellence. For example, Juran understood that, until recently, healthcare leaders had only a vague understanding of the scope, magnitude, implications, and ramifications of medication administration errors in the process of giving drugs to patients. Even though hospitals required nurses to report medication errors promptly, nurses had learned that when they made such reports, they were often subjected to unwarranted blame.

QUALITY IS FREE

Phillip Crosby coined this quality mantra to justify significant QM resource commitment in healthcare provider organizations:

"Quality is free. It's not a gift, it is free. What costs money is not quality things . . . , but rather all those actions that involve *not* doing jobs right the first time."

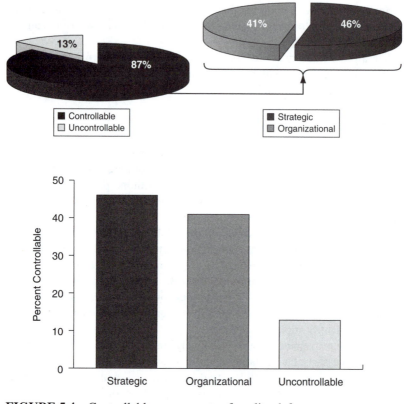

FIGURE 5.4   Controllable components of quality defects.

Crosby viewed quality as "conformance to requirements," with an organizational goal to "satisfy patient requirements first, last, and always." He advocated digital transformation of systems to improve quality of care delivery processes and applications. Transformation requires focus on prevention that recognizes that prevention requires a comprehensive understanding of processes to identify and remediate problems. Crosby advocated "zero defects" as an ultimate quality goal with staff and management throughout a provider organization who is constantly striving to achieve this goal.

Crosby taught that an ideal quality measure is the "cost of quality" with two components:

- *Price of nonconformance*, including internal failure costs, such as reinspection, retesting, scrap, rework, repairs, and lost production, and external costs, such as legal services, liability, damage claims, replacement, and lost customers. Crosby estimated that nonconformance costs likely represent 25% to 30% of organization costs.

- *Price of conformance*, including education, training, and prevention costs as well as inspection and testing. These costs are minimized in provider organizations by focusing on process improvement, error-cause removal, employee training and retraining, management leadership, and organization-wide quality awareness.

CAUSE AND EFFECT

Kaoru Ishikawa is known and credited for the development of the fishbone diagram, also called the Ishikawa diagram (see Chapter 2). He also developed and used quality control circles.

Ishikawa has been considered a quality control pioneer. His pragmatic approach and straightforward methods are well suited for healthcare provider organizations challenged by rapid change while simultaneously undertaking pervasive digital transformation.

These are key quality control principles for which Ishikawa is best known:

- *Pinpoint* aspects of quality that *paying* customers (i.e., patients, employers, insurance companies, and physicians) really want
- *Move* from inspection-based programs to a patient-centric process-oriented focus, establishing and administering a comprehensive quality control program with both vertical and cross-functional control
- *Use* basic statistical tools (i.e., cause and effect diagrams, Pareto analyses, histograms, etc.) to pinpoint and root out underlying error sources (i.e., those that prevent these errors from recurring)

BE THE BEST

> Benchmarking is a straightforward structured process used to develop new perspectives on care delivery processes and systems, patient needs, or requirements of customers

Tools such as **benchmarking** are often used to prudently and pragmatically measure credibility. Healthcare provider organizations use benchmarking to improve work processes and achieve these objectives by identifying, analyzing, and emulating best practices used inside and outside of healthcare organizations.

As an improvement team identifies a process to be improved, team members need to compare their process performance to similar processes in organizations recognized for "world class" performance and then establish this level of performance as a benchmark to meet and exceed. These methods can be studied to find out why they work so well in other organizations. These techniques can then be adopted, adapted, or emulated.

- *Look* at standard practices from a different perspective
- *Identify* performance goals for excellence
- *Facilitate* kaizen and breakthrough process improvement
- *Measure* then *monitor* progress toward excellence
- *Recognize, analyze,* and *emulate* best practices of quality leaders, regardless of industry (e.g., hospitals, ambulatory care centers, and hotels), that deliver comparable services or offer different services with common critical processes

In other industries, competitive benchmarking is commonly used to analyze competitors' products or services. Xerox Corporation is credited as having pioneered benchmarking techniques when they were interested in evaluating manufacturing costs. Competitors' products were dismantled, analyzed, and ultimately reengineered by Xerox to reduce manufacturing costs, improve quality, and include desirable functions and features. Early results of these early benchmarking studies demonstrated that Xerox's competitors were selling products at a price comparable with Xerox's manufacturing cost. Based on these initial successful study results, Xerox introduced enterprise-wide benchmarking. The rest, as they say, is history.

George Labovitz, an early leader in the growth of continuous process improvement in health care, articulated this now classic definition of benchmarking:

"A structured process for gaining new perspectives on the needs of patients and other customers. The objective in benchmarking in provider organizations is to improve work processes by identifying, measuring, and emulating best practices of service organizations inside and outside the healthcare industry."

As he explained, this approach recognizes an important strategy for achieving quality. To be the best, compare yourself with the best. Being the best in a community may not be very difficult, but striving to become the very best challenges everyone with opportunities for personal and professional growth.

Benchmarking has been used extensively in early productivity management system development to compare performance against similar providers. These benchmarking concepts and comparative analyses have been easier to understand and implement in organizations already using a productivity management system.

Experienced managers in these organizations understand these basic concepts (you can't manage what you don't measure). Benchmarks facilitate organization-wide adoption of continuous process improvement. A fundamental understanding of these concepts empowers providers in learning about organizations to continually strive to improve daily operations.

For example, when a provider organization develops a new program or service, evaluation team members may study other facilities, including those regarded as the best in providing those services. By benchmarking, team members are able to study how these healthcare organizations have developed and implemented similar programs and services.

This discussion is expanded further in Chapter 9 as productivity measurement and performance management approaches are introduced in the context of staffing and productivity benchmarking metrics.

SUMMARY

This chapter introduced QM terminology, tools, techniques, and concepts and explained how they are applicable in healthcare provider organizations.

Fundamental concepts and content focused on

- Definitions of quality
- QM, BPR, and Six Sigma
- Quality pioneers
- Conformance and nonconformance costs of quality
- Benchmarking

CHAPTER QUESTIONS

These questions reinforce student understanding, learning, and retention while stimulating class discussion:

1. Explain why there are different definitions for quality.
2. Who are considered the leading QM pioneers?
3. What is meant by the terms *conformance* and *nonconformance costs of quality*?
4. Why do benchmarking?

ADDITIONAL RESOURCES

These references are recommended for additional reading and more comprehensive content beyond the scope of this book.

Barry, R., Murcko, A., Brubaker, C. (2002). The Six Sigma Book for Healthcare. Chicago: Health Administration Press.

Bassard, M., Ritter, D. (1994). The Memory Jogger: A Pocket Guide of Tools for Continuous Improvement and Effective Planning. Salem, NH: Goal/QPC.

Caldwell, C. (1998). The Handbook for Managing Change in Health Care. Milwaukee, WI: Quality Press.

Crosby, P. (1979). Quality Is Free. New York: McGraw-Hill.

Deming, W. E. (1986). Out of Crisis. Boston: MIT Press.

Griffith, J., White, K. (2002). The Well-Managed Healthcare Organization. Chicago: Health Administration Press.

Herzlinger, R. (1997). Market-Driven Health Care: Who Wins, Who Loses in the Transformation of America's Largest Service Industry. Reading, MA: Perseus Books.

Ishikaw, K. (1985). Cause and Effect: The Japanese Way. Englewood Cliffs, NJ: Prentice-Hall.

Juran, J. M., Godrey, A. B. (1999). What Is Quality Control? New York: McGraw-Hill.

Labovitz, G. (1997). The Power of Alignment. Billerica, MA: Organization Dynamics.

Larson, J. (2001). Management Engineering. Chicago: Healthcare Information and Management Systems Society.

Longest, Jr., B., Rakich, J., Darr, K. (2004). Managing Health Services Organizations and Systems. Baltimore, MD: Health Professions Press.

Seidel, L., Gorsky, R., Lewis, J. (1995). Applied Quantitative Methods for Health Services Management. Baltimore, MD: Health Professions Press.

Wan, T. (1995). Analysis and Evaluation of Health Care Systems: An Integrated Approach to Managerial Decision Making. Baltimore, MD: Health Professions Press.

CHAPTER 6

Process Redesign Strategies

This chapter introduces process redesign strategies as BPR, focusing on

- BPR definition and terminology
- Differentiation of QM continuous process improvement, BPR concepts, and Six Sigma initiatives
- Substantial "order of magnitude" improvements
- Classic works likening contemporary health care to a focused factory

Hammer and Champy's classic BPR definition was articulated in *Reengineering the Corporation* as the "Fundamental rethinking and radical redesign of business processes as required to achieve dramatic improvements in critical and contemporary measures of performance, such as cost, quality, service, and speed."

This chapter highlights key BPR themes and compares BPR with other less rigorous process improvement approaches that are best used for processes deemed worthy of only limited remediation effort and resource investment. Attributes of a focused factory are described as competence that is derived from simplicity and repetition.

Champy, Hammer, Herzlinger, Skinner, and other pioneering transformationalists view classic BPR as popularized in the late 20th century as a contemporaneous variant of QM and continuous process improvement as embraced by JCAHO (previously discussed in Chapter 5). Therefore an underlying premise is that QM and continuous process improvement, as mandated for enterprise-wide implementation by JCAHO, presume that a "broken process" can and should be repaired with relatively limited intervention, using those techniques.

Alternatively, *BPR is justified upon acknowledgment that an existing process is so broken that it cannot and should not be just superficially "improved" as a long-term solution.* As such, BPR initiatives obligate a healthcare provider to break down existing process segments into discrete elemental tasks and then redesign task sequences into coherent business processes. BPR capitalizes on state-of-the-art ITs in addition to, or instead of, less invasive techniques associated with quality improvement initiatives.

In a traditional QM continuous process improvement initiative, a breakthrough is a potential yet rarely achieved expectation. Rather, a continuous, iterative, and incremental improvement, as expressed by the Japanese term "kaizen," is a more realistic outcome. As an alternative to kaizen, a breakthrough, by definition, requires a substantial investment in IT and organizational resources to achieve a higher level of increased process consistency, quality, and less variant performance than BPR necessarily drives to breakthrough success.

BPR initiatives, rather than QM projects, are much more likely to achieve effective digital transformation of targeted processes. It is essential that senior leadership understands this critical outcome expectation difference between QM and BPR. This basic understanding is very important as providers are challenged by a fast-paced increasingly competitive healthcare marketplace. This marketplace demands quicker, safer, and higher quality care delivery at a persistently lower cost. How a provider responds to these demands with an approach yielding higher outcome expectations determines whether an organization thrives or even survives through this decade.

Hammer, Champy, and other BPR advocates articulated these resonating BPR themes:

- *Combine* multiple jobs into one.
- *Empower* workers to make their own decisions.
- *Perform* process steps in a natural order.
- *Perform* work in the most sensible location.
- *Reduce* checks and controls.
- *Minimize* redundant reconciliation.
- *Provide* case managers as single patient-centric contacts and advocates.
- *Consider* centralized, decentralized, or hybrid operations for processes requiring multiple versions or operating in differing environments.

These contemporary "high tech, high touch" themes are technology dependent and embody traditional work simplification techniques that are described in Chapter 8.

BPR analyses are analogous to differential diagnosis used by clinicians (i.e., viewed from a perspective of symptoms versus diseases). Extensive information exchange, data redundancy, and rekeying are symptoms that reflect an organizational disease of arbitrary fragmentation of a natural process. Similarly, processing related to inventory buffers are symptoms that reflect a systemic latent disease with imbalanced ambivalence to coping with uncertainties.

A high ratio of checking and control to value-added activities reflects systemic fragmentation, rework, and iterative burdens. Any complex system with a high checking-to-control ratio demonstrates inadequate feedback along chains, exceptions, and special cases. These symptoms illustrate progressive pervasive administration and unnecessary unproductive bureaucratic complexity that adds little if any value and demonstrates an unhealthy accretion upon what was once an elegantly simple delivery infrastructure.

Reengineering teams learn a great deal about processes while diagnosing current process problems but must not focus on only fixing them. A BPR team can only be successful when they recognize and acknowledge that a legacy process requires so much fixing only to yield marginal benefit and therefore does not warrant any additional effort. BPR teams do not look for marginal benefits but rather for order-of-magnitude improvements. Simply fixing old processes is rarely good enough, especially for mission critical and strategically vital processes. BPR teams analyze existing processes to learn and understand those critical components that contribute most (i.e., add value) to overall process performance. As team members gain more knowledge and begin to understand true objectives of each process, they become increasingly effective at process redesign.

Following are time-tested recommendations that encourage an expeditious and highly energized organizational approach to design and execute significant change at each process level. These objectives embody valuable strategic principles and useful tactical guidelines that increase the probability of a reengineering team's success:

- *Involve* as few people as possible in the performance of each process.
- *Use* someone other than a subject-matter expert to lead the effort to redesign a process.
- *Recognize* that being an outsider helps (e.g., an effective project manager or team leader does not need to know much about an existing process).
- *View* each process from a patient's perspective.
- *Discard* preconceived notions.
- *Redesign* each process by using deliberate, cogent, and collaborative team-driven initiatives guided by clearly articulated objectives.
- *Emphasize* that it is not difficult to identify and develop great ideas.
- *Recognize* that process redesign, although sometimes painful, is no less important and organizationally rewarding.
- *Develop* failure strategies, recognizing that significant lessons are learned by experience and through understanding of how and why previous BPR projects failed.

Alternatively, these examples are time tested failure strategies to be avoided:

- *Trying* to fix rather than change a process
- *Focusing* on business processes and ignoring everything except process redesign
- *Concentrating* exclusively on design, neglecting staff values and beliefs, while accepting only limited results
- *Quitting* too early or placing prior constraints on problem definition and scope of a reengineering project
- *Tolerating* corporate cultures and management attitudes that inhibit reengineering efforts, while burying BPR in mundane corporate agendas that dissipate energy across too many initiatives
- *Trying* to make reengineering happen from the bottom up
- *Failing* to distinguish reengineering from other process improvement programs
- *Assigning* someone who does not understand reengineering to lead initiatives
- *Attempting* to reengineer critical processes as a senior leader is departing or approaching retirement
- *Relying* on resources not dedicated to reengineering
- *Attempting* to achieve real change without making anybody unhappy
- *Retreating* as reengineering changes encounter resistance, thereby prolonging the BPR process

Classic writings by Hammer and Champy include detailed case studies of these failure strategies. Serious BPR practitioners and aspiring digital transformationalists should carefully study these lessons as well as relevant portions of Herzlinger's *Market-Driven Health Care: Who Wins, Who Loses in a Digital Transformation of America's Largest Service Industry?*

Herzlinger teaches specific lessons of a broad scope, such as "do not integrate vertically to protect a faltering business" and "focus, focus, focus." Herzlinger often refers to Skinner's focused factory with simplicity and repetition propagating competence. Herzlinger's work likens successful healthcare organizations to "factories" that focus on a narrow product mix for a particular market niche and thereby outperform any conventional facility with a broader mission.

SUMMARY

This chapter presented important terminology, tools, techniques, and concepts that described how and when BPR is applicable in healthcare provider organizations.

Fundamental concepts and content focused on

- BPR definition and terminology required for a fundamental rethinking and radical redesign of business process
- Differentiation of BPR themes of QM projects and Six Sigma initiatives
- Expectations for order of magnitude improvement
- Classics likening contemporary healthcare to a focused factory

CHAPTER QUESTIONS

These questions reinforce student understanding, learning, and retention while stimulating class discussion:

1. Define BPR.
2. Differentiate between the BPR themes of QM projects and Six Sigma initiatives.
3. What is meant by order of magnitude improvement?

ADDITIONAL RESOURCES

These references are recommended for additional reading and more comprehensive content beyond the scope of this book.

Barry, R., Murcko, A., Brubaker, C. (2002). The Six Sigma Book for Healthcare. Chicago: Health Administration Press.

Bassard, M., Ritter, D. (1994). The Memory Jogger: A Pocket Guide of Tools for Continuous Improvement and Effective Planning. Salem, NH: Goal/QPC.

Hammer, M., Champy, T. (2001). Re-Engineering the Corporation. New York: Harper Collins Publishers.

Herzlinger, R. (1997). Market-Driven Health Care: Who Wins, Who Loses in the Transformation of America's Largest Service Industry. Reading, MA: Perseus Books.

Larson, J. (2001). Management Engineering. Chicago: Healthcare Information and Management Systems Society.

Wan, T. (1995). Analysis and Evaluation of Health Care Systems: An Integrated Approach to Managerial Decision Making. Baltimore, MD: Health Professions Press.

CHAPTER 7

Transformational Strategies for Tactical Project Management

This chapter highlights digital transformation strategies by focusing on tactical project management and recently successful transformation achievements in patient care.

Fundamental concepts and content include

- Project management control and evaluation requirements
- Tactical use of scheduling tools and critical path analysis
- Work breakdown structure
- Performance improvement expectations
- Examples of successfully transformed provider organizations

Successful transformations are being driven by leaders who actively initiate and manage enterprise-wide change. These successes reflect a variety of complimentary themes.

Progressive, pragmatic, organizational leaders have common attributes, such as demonstrating adoption and forward-thinking managerial innovation. As has been proven in other successfully transformed service industries, such as banking, project management tools and related tactical techniques enable provider organizations to achieve successful process redesign. When embraced and supported by leaders, this approach provides a thematic foundation upon which sustainable change with deliberate discipline and structure is built.

Each of these tools and techniques had manufacturing sector origins. They were then emulated within service organizations and recently by healthcare providers. These tools and techniques are simply classic industrial engineering and project management methodologies that have been adapted for unique characteristics of healthcare delivery.

Society, employers, government, payers, and especially large healthcare plans and providers have expressed increasing concern about limited organization focus on care delivery. Performance characteristics' efficiency, and effectiveness issues such as quality, cost, availability, and competitiveness, require more senior management attention and organization-wide resource allocation. In response, improved facility designs, especially trained staff, specialized equipment, instrumentation, systems, and procedures, are concentrated on more streamlined tasks for each unique group of patients. In these concentrated niches of expertise, astute, innovative, and competitive providers accomplish key tasks that are more effectively targeted at strategic mission-driven requirements. In these islands of excellence, delivery quality is higher and costs are lower than those of conventional providers.

Table 7.1 summarizes opportunities to improve quality and increase provider productivity while reducing workload and costs. These expected outcomes of

TABLE 7.1   Performance Improvement Expectations

Improve Labor Effectiveness Increase Personnel Efficiency	Improve Nonlabor Utilization Decrease Supply Consumption
• Analyze, automate processes through accelerated digital transformation	• Conduct waste analysis
• Enhance scheduling and real-time staffing analyses to level	• Evaluate usage rate per procedure
	• Breakage
• Educate management and supervisors in time management, work simplification, process improvement, and worksite redesign	• Pilferage
	• Obsolescence
• Update equipment, information systems, and technology to optimize staffing proficiency, mix, levels, and capabilities	• Evaluate inventory level by use analysis
• Increase outputs, not inputs, thereby reducing unit costs and improving proficiency with education and training	
• Incorporate incentives, bonuses and as penalty clauses for contracted services	

digital transformation of delivery processes yield positive impacts on provider and organization performance.

Recent influential studies (e.g., *To Err Is Human, Crossing the Quality Chasm?*) are critical of the quality of care in America's healthcare delivery system, characterizing current processes as woefully inadequate, with much improvement required. These examples highlight progressive organizations that are confronting these challenges with digital transformation tools (e.g., QM, BPR, Six Sigma initiatives) that improve care quality while reducing care delivery cost.

These organizations voluntarily participated in the CMS pilot program that tested outcomes for "pay for performance" outcome, achieving top-tier performance in all care delivery standards:

- *Deaconess Hospital* in Indiana reduced expected inpatient mortality rates by more than 10% below those achieved in comparable facilities nationally. This regional trauma center performs better than all CMS core metrics for acute myocardial infarction, congestive heart failure, and community-acquired pneumonia. An internal measure of patient arrival to perfusion time for emergency cardiac admissions was reduced to levels that were substantially better than American College of Cardiology recommendations.
- *Hackensack University Medical Center* in New Jersey has steadily improved quality and demonstrated leading-edge performance by redesigning care delivery processes.
- *McLeod Regional Medical Center* in South Carolina dramatically reduced medication-related patient injuries to increase patient safety and improve care quality and simultaneously reduce operating costs.

This CMS pilot test has since been adopted and tied to reimbursement models for all acute care hospitals.

America's largest healthcare provider, the Department of Veterans Affairs (VA), has significantly improved quality and controlled costs. An independent and widely respected nonprofit research organization compared patient care in VA facilities to care provided by similar facilities outside the VA system. This organization's study concluded that VA patients received recommended care 15% more often than patients served by non-VA providers. Specifically, the Rand Corporation found that

- VA patients received 67% of recommended care
- Patients treated in non-VA facilities received only 51% of recommended services

The Rand Corporation report encourages other providers to follow the pioneering VA's digital transformation approach. These approaches included the improved use of IT, electronic health records and prescriptions instead of paper, and automated performance tracking.

Effective transformational projects demonstrated by these examples require deliberate planning, disciplined strategy, and tactical deployment structure. These tactics incorporate both the art and science of dynamic situational decision-making focused on project scope, schedules, and costs to produce effective high-quality results.

Project teams achieve these objectives, with each team consistently focused on digital transformation of mission-critical processes. Necessary improvement of healthcare delivery processes are often centered around deliberate deployment of "disruptive technologies." To successfully achieve desired outcomes in initiatives of this magnitude, project management necessarily requires careful and thoughtful planning, scheduling, and control of project activities.

Most project management emphasis is devoted to essential tasks of planning, scheduling, and controlling. Managing human behaviors of both staff-sensitive and patient-centric aspects are important. Effective human resource management is essential to ensure that appropriate personnel with requisite skills and management competencies are in the right place at an appropriate time.

THE PROJECT MANAGEMENT PROCESS

The Project Management Institute is a professional association for project managers.

This organization describes a project management process that incorporates these major phases:

- Initiation
- Planning
- Scheduling
- Risk Assessment and Management
- Control
- Evaluation

Initiation

In this first phase a project's scope is established and the addressable problem(s) with care delivery processes are agreed upon.

Planning

This phase is devoted to developing a project definition that is clearly and succinctly articulated, including any associated constraints. For example, a project plan is a document that summarizes responses to each of these questions for each task:

- *What* must be done and *why*?
- *Who* should be assigned to the project team?
- *How* will the project be organized and performed?
- *When* must the project be completed?
- *How* much is the project expected to cost?
- *What* resources are needed?

Scheduling

In this phase the project manager leads assigned team members through anticipated work assignments to solve defined problem(s) as identified in earlier phases.

By using a generic project plan developed in previous phases, the project manager develops an even more detailed project work plan. This document must be developed and agreed on by the entire team before any project work begins. This document must be detailed enough so that each task to be completed is described in a step-by-step format.

Sufficient time must be devoted to this phase of a project's life cycle to increase the likelihood of project success. In this context, project success is defined as having met expectations documented in the initial phase. This approach results in the effective use of resources at appropriate times as a project is conceptualized, planned, defined, designed, implemented, evaluated, and ultimately completed.

A work plan is developed during this phase that consists of defined tasks in a disciplined and focused manner to avoid unforeseen overlap among tasks. Task leaders are assigned the responsibility to monitor progress and report status for each task and subtask at regularly scheduled meetings or reporting periods.

Target dates are necessary to guide task leaders and to ensure logical task sequencing and performance. Deliverables are described as individual and team work products of this work breakdown structure (WBS), including requirements for achievement that meet project objectives. Some deliverables are time sensitive, requiring careful planning and effective use of resources to meet project milestones.

A "best practice" used to develop accurate and achievable WBSs is a technique called work decomposition. Work decomposition requires that

- Each task is unambiguous
- Task work elements are only those related to that task
- Task work elements are performed by the same team member(s)
- Team members who perform the work should participate in developing this WBS

Lessons learned from unsuccessful projects inevitably reflect missing or ineffectively developed WBSs. For example, common shortfalls include

- Insufficient time allocation
- Inadequate resource allocation
- Poor communication during project planning and execution

Upon completion of the project work plan, including a detailed WBS, a project schedule is prepared as tasks and subtasks are matched with a calendar that spans the anticipated project duration. Effective project management results from an accurate project schedule that is developed and executed as agreed on by all team members.

This scheduling process is a necessary validation to ensure that project objectives and deadlines are achievable as planned. A project schedule is necessary to meet project deadlines and to identify a project's *critical path*. Figure 7.1 is an example of a critical path on a network diagram.

Network diagrams are used to depict critical and sometimes complicated task relationships; for example, task A is performed before task B, whereas tasks B and C start simultaneously with task D, which cannot begin until tasks A and C are completed. Such relationships are best displayed as network diagrams.

Networking Diagramming

Figure 7.1 is an example of a "high-level" network diagram, depicting task relationships as well as a critical path for this generic project's life cycle. The project's critical path is highlighted.

Although a WBS is essential to effective project planning, management, and execution, WBS development often occurs simultaneously with staffing and sequencing tasks. For example, if projected earliest start to latest finish time estimates for WBS development include 2 days of float time, WBS development is unlikely to be on the project's critical path if all work is completed as scheduled. However, if a WBS takes 3 days longer to complete than anticipated, then a modified network diagram would show WBS development as a critical task on the project's critical path.

Network diagrams include appropriate descriptive information (e.g., task name, start and finish dates, duration, percentage of completion, etc.). Lines between tasks describe task and subtask sequences scheduled for completion. Critical path tasks are highlighted with a set of tasks that must be completed as scheduled to complete the project on time. Critical paths are determined by inspecting simple project network diagrams or by using complex algorithms as required for more complicated projects. Although beyond the scope of this chapter, commercially

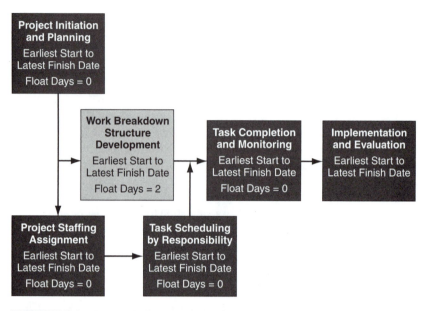

FIGURE 7.1   Network diagram with critical path.

available project management software automatically calculates and highlights critical paths. Network diagrams that depict a project's critical path are frequently called a "project map."

Analysis of a network diagram determines a project's critical path at any point in time and is derived from these intrinsic task properties:

- Earliest start date
- Latest start date
- Earliest finish date
- Latest finish date
- Available float time (i.e., permissible "slack" or slippage of a task's completion without significant impact project scheduling)

Critical tasks are those determined to *not have any float time*. Therefore a path from project start to project finish that includes all critical tasks in the least time possible is a critical path.

Determination of a project's critical path(s) is essential information for the project manager to plan and control the project. Understanding the nature and flexibility of each task is vital to focus on those critical tasks that, if delayed, will result in unacceptable slippage in a project's schedule. There may be more than one critical path, depending on project scheduling and variability of each task's completion.

Each critical path is a unique sequence of tasks that must be completed so that an overall project schedule is maintained and project objectives are achieved as anticipated. In most projects only some tasks are on the critical path, whereas many tasks may not be on the critical path. In other words, task delays on the critical path are those that directly impact project deadlines.

Conversely, delays for tasks that are not on the critical path will not affect the project's completion deadline. However, this should not be interpreted to mean that a "noncritical" task can be ignored. If a noncritical task is delayed long enough, it becomes part of the project's critical path.

Gantt Charts

Gantt charts and network diagrams are the most important tools and techniques used to develop and maintain a project schedule. Both are necessary to understand priority relationships among and between tasks.

A **Gantt chart** is a special type of bar graph with time displayed horizontally and tasks shown vertically on each respective axis.

Figures 7.2 and 7.3 are examples of Gantt chart formats used in healthcare project planning.

In these figures tasks A through J represent task names on each vertical axis. Each example shows various impacts on a project schedule.

Similarly, Figures 7.4 and 7.5 are example formats used by project managers to monitor task status and compare and report planned and actual task duration.

Tasks A through J depict task progress against time at a specific point in time (e.g., a project status reporting date).

As Figures 7.2 through Figure 7.5 illustrate, Gantt charts are excellent tools to depict, analyze, and report task schedules. While a project is underway, they are used to report task progress and completion status to executive sponsors, project managers, and team members. All project stakeholders need to understand and appreciate critical relationships among and between tasks. Reporting of this type is essential, especially during initial project planning and then periodically throughout a project life cycle.

Risk Assessment and Management

Upon completion of a project plan, the project manager must assess risks associated with each task. For each task as any risk is identified a mitigation strategy

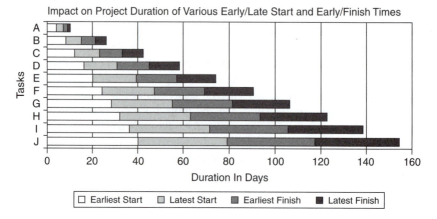

FIGURE 7.2   Project planning using Gantt chart.

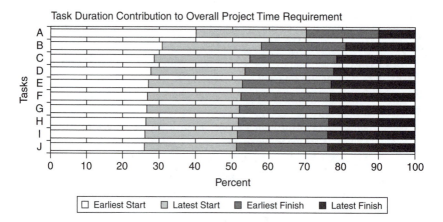

FIGURE 7.3   Potential impacts of task time duration using Gantt chart.

should be developed. Often, risk is only variable in terms of labor or materials and their associated cost. Typically, adjusting work estimates mitigates risk with task-by-task adjustments accumulated for a project.

Control

Control is an important aspect of project management because it is required to effectively manage resources and to achieve expected high-quality results as expe-

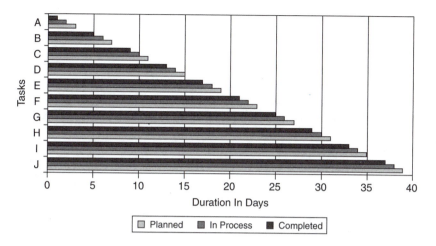

FIGURE 7.4   Project management and completion status using Gantt chart.

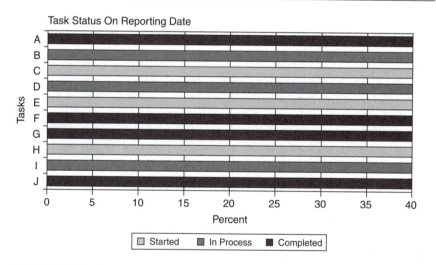

FIGURE 7.5   Gantt chart reporting task completion status.

ditiously and as cost-effectively as possible. Put another way, control reinforces management of project resources so that the project is completed within scope, on schedule, and within budgetary constraints.

Project control includes those activities required to compare progress of each critical task with the project plan to identify necessary actions that correct deviations in a timely manner. This phase parallels execution and requires consistent, and persistent project status assessment by repeatedly asking "Is the task on target?" If not, the project manager must develop and initiate the required action(s) to complete the project as planned.

Control is best accomplished when all project resources are included as active participants in a project's control cycle.

Project managers establish, maintain, and sustain control by

- *Clarifying* objectives for each team member
- *Negotiating* a personal work plan for each team member
- *Ensuring* that each team member has appropriate and can demonstrate requisite competencies
- *Providing* and *soliciting* feedback to and from team members throughout a project control cycle
- *Defining* individual team member authority to make real-time corrections within their area(s) of responsibility when confronted with a deviation from planned tasks

Unless a control system includes corrective action requirements it is *not* a control system, merely a monitoring system.

Recognizing that a variety of tools support differing approaches to project control, many of which are computer, network, or Internet driven, the core requirement remains that team members must provide data to the project manager in a timely, structured, and succinct manner. Some applications are easily administered by voice or video conference that includes associated audio-video documentation and archival capability. Others may be accomplished with dialogue among and between team members and the project manager. Regardless of media and vehicle, frequent and direct dialogue between the project manager and each team member is critical. Written status reports are useful but should not replace dialogue.

Control systems should only require vital information that can be collected and reported as painlessly as possible. Project managers should design and adopt a project control system, minimizing reporting burdens placed on team members. Team members have been tasked to produce work, *not* reports. Many staff project team members are assigned to a project(s) as collateral duty while retaining an ongoing responsibility for full-time organizational responsibilities.

Evaluation

A project manager should continually assess progress in terms of current status, anticipated future status, critical tasks status, risk assessment, and lessons learned.

Based on data provided by team members during a project's entire life cycle, project status should be frequently communicated to all team members and stakeholders. Reporting frequency and publication of project status reports should be driven by project complexity and organizational culture.

Although many process redesign solutions require some sort of technology-based support, many can be effectively addressed by astute hands-on guidance led by senior management action.

Fundamental changes that digitally transform care delivery processes do not necessarily require high-tech solutions. Rather simple insightful inquiry, careful observation, critical and careful analysis, coupled with thoughtful, well-designed, and effectively implemented solutions is ideal.

Clinicians need time and other resources to ensure that safe and effective care is delivered as patients flow through provider organizations. Patient diagnostics and treatment has to be delivered in optimal settings so that patients are satisfied customers who receive high-quality cost-effective care that meets each individual's unique needs. Care providers need to be more focused on effective patient care and not frustrated by poor patient and process flow that inevitably leads to subpar clinical outcomes. Project management of digital transformation initiatives is both a strategic and tactical requirement to achieve desired outcomes. Action-oriented leadership requires that top executives routinely demonstrate involvement by

- *Talking* to patients waiting to be treated and also after treatment to understand provider performance and patients' expectations compared with their experiences
- *Visiting* patient care settings (e.g., emergency department or outpatient diagnostic centers) and carefully observing patient routing and delivery settings that typical patients experience, then ask and document answers to questions such as
  - Are waiting rooms clean, patient and family friendly, and conducive to expectations of high-quality care delivery?
  - Are patients acknowledged upon arrival by qualified triage nursing staff?
  - Are patients and families kept informed and courteously treated?
  - What are patients and staff doing while waiting?
  - Are staff efficiently engaged in hands-on care or unproductively idle?
- *Meeting* with physicians, nurses, and other clinical staff in spontaneous discussions or town meetings in all departments on all shifts, asking if they feel fulfilled as they accomplish job requirements
- *Communicating* a constant need for operational change to achieve mission and vision, using digital transformation to deliver better care from improved patient and process flow

SUMMARY

Project management terminology, tools, techniques, and concepts were discussed. Attributes of successful digital transformation projects in effective provider organizations are highlighted.

Fundamental concepts and content included

- Project management control and evaluation requirements
- Tactical use of scheduling tools and critical path analysis
- WBS
- Performance improvement expectations
- Examples of successfully transformed healthcare provider organizations

CHAPTER QUESTIONS

These questions reinforce student understanding, learning, and retention while stimulating class discussion:

1. How are project planning and management requirements different?
2. What is meant by WBS?
3. Discuss a successfully transformed example.

ADDITIONAL RESOURCES

These references are recommended for additional reading and more comprehensive content beyond the scope of this book.

Bassard, M., Ritter, D. (1994). The Memory Jogger: A Pocket Guide of Tools for Continuous Improvement and Effective Planning. Salem, NH: Goal/QPC.

Kohn, L., Corrigan, J., and Donaldson, M. (2000). To Err Is Human. National Academy Press, Washington, D.C.

Kohn, L., Corrigan, J., Donaldson, M. (2000). Crossing the Quality Chasm: A New Healthcare System for the 21st Century. National Academy Press, Washington, D.C.

Larson, J. (2001). Management Engineering. Chicago: Healthcare Information and Management Systems Society.

Martin, P., Tate, K. (1997). Project Management Memory Jogger: A Pocket Guide for Project Teams. Salem, NH: Goal/QPC.

Veney, J., Kaluzny, A. (1998). Evaluation and Decision Making for Health Services. Chicago: Health Administration Press.

Wan, T. (1995). Analysis and Evaluation of Health Care Systems: An Integrated Approach to Managerial Decision Making. Baltimore, MD: Health Professions Press.

CHAPTER 8

Tactical Work Breakdown and Workload Analysis

This chapter introduces work breakdown and workload analysis with a focus on these key concepts:

- Work simplification objectives and approaches
- Work distribution
- Why techniques
- Flow process analysis and documentation
- Horizontal flow analysis
- Time flow analysis
- Job sequencing

Focus on "working smarter, not harder." This straightforward cliché aptly describes tools and techniques described in this chapter. Most experts admit that these tools are little more than "an organized application of common sense."

WORK SIMPLIFICATION

Classic management science and industrial engineering concepts were applied at a managerial or supervisory level. More recently, these techniques have been embodied in team-driven QM and process reengineering initiatives.

Work simplification objectives reflect an unbiased evaluation of activities, using two-way communication and collaboration, teamwork among employees at all organizational levels, a consultative approach to problem identification, and resolution as well as a timely recognition of contribution. These simple yet powerful

111

techniques are designed to tap many creative minds and generate productive quality improvement and cost-reduction ideas otherwise untapped in staff throughout an organization. Such insightful ideas rarely get communicated to decision-makers and unfortunately remain to stagnate.

This approach involves eight fundamental steps to process improvement through work simplification:

1. *Select* processes or situations requiring improvement of actionable high-priority problems characterized by excessive workloads, taking too much work home, backlogs, filled "in" baskets, excessive overtime, or high labor costs for simple tasks. Organizations typically start with a simple process where the probability of success is high, reserving long-standing more difficult problems, applying this approach to complex systems after basic techniques have been mastered. Work simplification practitioners must appreciate that each job has three fundamental parts: getting ready, doing task(s), and cleanup and breakdown of required materials and facilities.

2. *Consult* all concerned participants associated with each process to improve cooperation and make changes easier to implement; focus on problems from different perspectives to identify potentially optimal solutions. Most solutions will not be those developed by the practitioner but rather will be directly identified or implied by those routinely doing the job.

3. *Collect* all relevant facts by focusing on what, where, when, why, and how. Use open-ended questioning techniques, initially rely on validation of existing policies, procedures, memoranda, job descriptions, time standards, work schedules, published statistics, and reports rather than starting with new or potentially redundant data by collecting all data from scratch. Team members should understand that using existing documents, policies, and procedures whenever possible is not only much easier, it is more cost-effective. Additionally, process participants are more likely to provide existing data or information if they do not have to write, replicate, or otherwise document responses to each question.

4. *Challenge* every detail and do not assume anything. Many systems were developed by others, and current staff may simply be perpetuating historical procedures without really understanding them. (See Figure 8.1 for a list of common questions to ask.)

5. *Consolidate* various options/combinations into defined alternatives that are presented in priority order. Do not present problems without solutions.

6. *Sell* first to process owners before administrative staff and then introduce proposals to process participants. Package the solution by discussing findings, conclusions, and recommendations with those who have to make solutions work. Small scale pilot tests of solutions are prudent before recommending large-scale implementations.

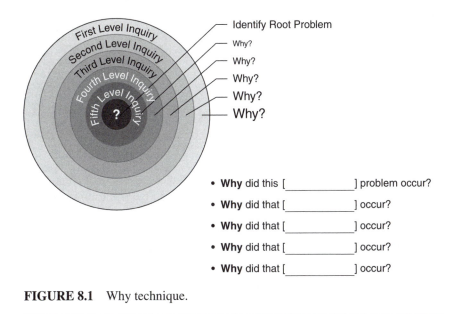

First Level Inquiry
Second Level Inquiry
Third Level Inquiry
Fourth Level Inquiry
Fifth Level Inquiry
?

Identify Root Problem
Why?
Why?
Why?
Why?
Why?

- **Why** did this [_____] problem occur?
- **Why** did that [_____] occur?
- **Why** did that [_____] occur?
- **Why** did that [_____] occur?
- **Why** did that [_____] occur?

FIGURE 8.1   Why technique.

7. *Encourage* constructive critical review and candid feedback to ensure that users understand and accept the solution. Conduct objective evaluations of outcome(s) periodically as appropriate. Follow through with recognition of process participants by formally acknowledging all those assisting in the effort.

8. *Identify* whether proposed actions have been implemented and desired results have been achieved. Determine whether the implementation schedule was followed. Measure benefits and quantify any negative side effects.

These simple yet powerful seven questions need to be asked and answered as often as possible in conjunction with each of these eight steps:

- *What* is being done?
- *Who* is doing it?
- *Where* is it being done?
- *How* is it being done?
- *When* is it being done?
- *Why* is it being done at all?
- *What* happens if not done?

- What?
- Who?
- Where?
- How?
- When?
- Why?
- What if not done?

Every detail of each job or task must next be challenged without exception or assumption. Many existing systems, processes, procedures, or jobs in healthcare organizations were frequently developed by others. Current staff may simply be perpetuating historical procedures without really understanding them or the reason they are doing them.

WHY TECHNIQUE

Frequently and almost predictably, when asked "why" a typical response is "we have always done it this way." As each existing task job or process is being explained by a process participant, team members are more likely to discover and better understand more detail if "why" is repeated several times. Figure 8.1 illustrates these simple but powerful "why techniques," are a tool often used.

As this current state of a process is being understood and documented, members should begin to identify likely opportunities to eliminate, combine, simplify, or improve each process step. This technique, although quite simple to use, is one of the most effective approaches to thoroughly document and understand current procedures, processes, or tasks:

- *Eliminate* tasks with a 100% potential savings yield expectation.
- *Combine* tasks with a 50% potential savings yield expectation.
- *Simplify* tasks with a 30% potential savings yield. expectation.
- *Improve* any task to yield at least a 20% savings.

Figure 8.2 shows how each of these work simplification options impact the setup, execution, and breakdown components of any task. Figure 8.3 highlights overall objectives of work simplification.

The most exciting redesign phase of a work simplification initiative should *not* be attempted until rigorous review and exhaustive analyses is completed to an appropriate level of detail. Team leaders or senior leadership sponsors of a work simplification initiative must constantly remind teams and team members *not* to

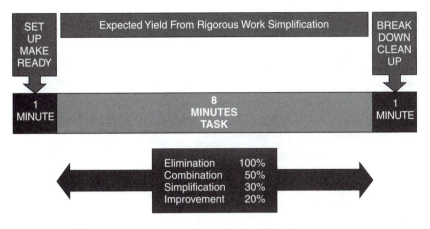

FIGURE 8.2 Expected yield from work simplification.

prejudge or presume to know a problem's root cause and prematurely design a solution.

Next, appropriate process improvement techniques identify, define, and explore various improvement options. Tools and techniques, include flowcharting, "imagineering," brainstorming, Pareto analyses, NGT, and affinity diagramming, complete current process documentation, problem identification, and analysis. Only then can developing and evaluating optional solutions be considered.

These versatile tools are also used to design, document, and evaluate options and ultimately propose a "future" solution while process redesign, reengineering, and improvement continue. Work simplification teams evaluate optional solutions after having gained a comprehensive understanding of potential savings in this evaluation and analytic phase.

As each process is thoroughly understood, expectations are less generic while becoming increasingly specific. Expectations are realistic and achievable if a process or task is previously analyzed from a work simplification perspective. By analyzing each task in every process, a team can eliminate, combine, simplify, and improve each step in all processes to identify potential solutions after exhaustive analyses of all options.

After team consensus for each conclusion is achieved, options are consolidated into defined alternatives and presented as team recommendations in priority order. A solution should be presented for each problem identified. When a problem remains unresolved, recommendations for additional analyses may accompany recommendations with a clarifying explanation (e.g., beyond project scope,

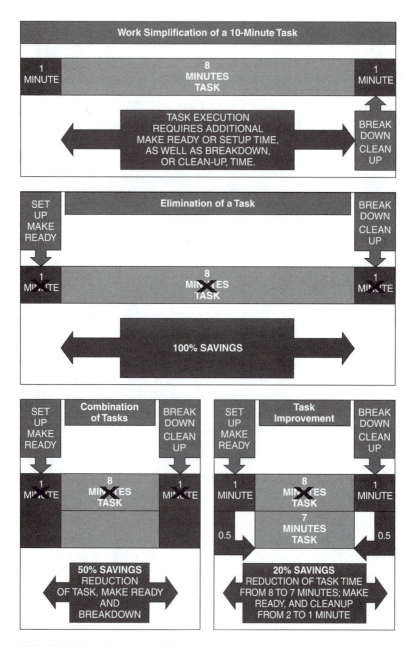

FIGURE 8.3   Work simplification objectives.

resources, time or funding). Before presentation, conclusions and recommendations should be reviewed with key process stakeholders. Team members should welcome constructive critical review and encourage candid feedback to ensure that process stakeholders, owners, and users understand and accept recommendations for change, acknowledge proposed process and technology solutions.

When process owners concur, study analyses, conclusions, and recommendations are ready for presentation. If process owners do not concur with a work simplification team's proposal(s), their rationale should be acknowledged, incorporated, and then presented with team recommendations to senior sponsors to build leadership support.

Whenever possible, pilot testing of each proposed solution is recommended before proceeding with a comprehensive implementation. Each recommendation should include an action plan to incorporate proposed responsibility and implementation timelines. A recommendation for an objective evaluation of implemented outcomes should also be included.

This post-implementation audit or evaluation should identify whether proposed recommendations were implemented and desired results achieved. This "after action" assessment should include an objective measure of cost and benefits and of unanticipated side effects or unintended consequences based on leadership direction and organization policy.

Implementation planning and scheduling should not begin until team recommendations are approved by organization leaders as team sponsors. Authorization to proceed with team recommendations may or may not include reasonable modification by senior leaders.

Depending on each project's unique nature and senior management's decision-making style, work simplification team members may or may not be asked to participate in a recommendation's implementation.

In conjunction with senior management and consistent with organizational protocol, recognition of work simplification team members and process participants should acknowledge those individuals who assisted with project data collection, analysis, development of conclusions, and presentation of recommendations.

WORK DISTRIBUTION ANALYSIS

Work distribution analysis identifies and develops relationships between assigned workload and resources that are allocated to accomplish assigned work. This technique enables comprehensive documentation of activities and contributions to achieve objectives from each departmental staff member.

Problems are identified and remediation options developed for specific problems by having department staff answer critical questions related to the current process:

- What work is accomplished?
- Who does this work?
- What contributions does each employee make to achieve departmental objectives?

Next, a work simplification analyst evaluates inefficiencies and staffing imbalances. Then, analyses of organizational structure and effectiveness are used to identify and further explore opportunities. Key steps include preparing lists of activities and tasks and analyzing all functions performed as identified and supervised. Identifying potentially redundant or inefficient work distribution is vital to assess potential for improved use of scarce and expensive labor resources.

Work distribution analysis involves design, facilitation, and collection of more detailed data using task lists. These lists are designed to include *all* identified tasks performed by each employee, including unproductive time. Because several individuals may perform more than one task, activities are listed in prioritized numerical sequence.

Work distribution analyses are usually based on a typical workweek. Typically, miscellaneous activities should not account for more than 15% to 20% of all activities identified. Defining task specificity and listing tasks in priority order are two important aspects of making data collection forms as easy as possible for departmental staff to complete as accurately and conveniently as possible. After departmental staff complete a week of data collection, a manager or supervisor should review and verify the "reasonableness" of each employee's data collection, compared with task lists and actual workload volume and hours worked during that week.

Figure 8.4 is a generic work distribution worksheet for a five-person workgroup (staff members A through D, including supervisor A). All members of this workgroup have indicated that everyone completes every task (tasks 1 through 5). Clearly, analysis of this work distribution warrants further study. Automated templates of this worksheet in spreadsheet workbooks facilitate both data collection and analysis.

Work simplification analysts reconcile activity and task lists by assigning activity numbers to each task. For reporting purposes a work distribution chart is created that depicts activity and task lists in descending order of importance within each activity, including estimated hours and volumes.

Either a Pareto diagram or a pie chart is ideal for analysis and presentation to focus and highlight

- What activities take significant time?
- Is there misdirected effort?
- Are skills properly used?
- Are employees doing too many unrelated tasks?

	Task 1	Task 2	Task 3	Task 4	Task 5
Unique Tasks →					
Staff Member A	Task 1 By Staff A	Task 2 By Staff A	Task 3 By Staff A	Task 4 By Staff A	Task 5 By Staff A
Staff Member B	Task 1 By Staff B	Task 2 By Staff B	Task 3 By Staff B	Task 4 By Staff B	Task 5 By Staff B
Staff Member C	Task 1 By Staff C	Task 2 By Staff C	Task 3 By Staff C	Task 4 By Staff C	Task 5 By Staff C
Staff Member D	Task 1 By Staff D	Task 2 By Staff D	Task 3 By Staff D	Task 4 By Staff D	Task 5 By Staff D
Supervisor A	Task 1 By Supervisor A	Task 2 By Supervisor A	Task 3 By Supervisor A	Task 4 By Supervisor A	Task 5 By Supervisor A

(Individual Staff Members ↓)

FIGURE 8.4   Work distribution worksheet.

- Are tasks too thinly spread?
- Is work distribution even?

FLOW PROCESS ANALYSIS

This technique is a variant of traditional flowcharting or imagineering that combines graphics and narrative to describe a single system, application, process, or procedure.

Employees' mental and physical activities or events associated with material processing can be tracked by using this tool. After choosing a function to be studied and subjects to be followed, initial steps of technique include

- Picking beginning and ending points
- Applying appropriate symbols for each operation (e.g., transportation, inspection, delay, and storage)
- Determining functions, quality, quantity, and distance to summarize overall process improvement potential

This technique is an excellent tool to present a before and after picture of significant process improvement. (Flowcharting techniques were previously presented and illustrated in Chapter 2.)

Figure 8.5 is a data collection worksheet that is useful when documenting workload distribution, work, and process flow. As with special flowcharting symbols, those depicted on the right columns may be customized to reflect unique specifications of each process, function, or application being studied. Each task is briefly described in sequence, including associated distances and time when relevant. Each task type and flow is indicated as a line drawn vertically through each symbol from the beginning to the end of each process. Each step is then documented in chronologic order from top to bottom or continued as necessary on subsequent worksheets. This tool is especially useful during staff interviews to capture workflow

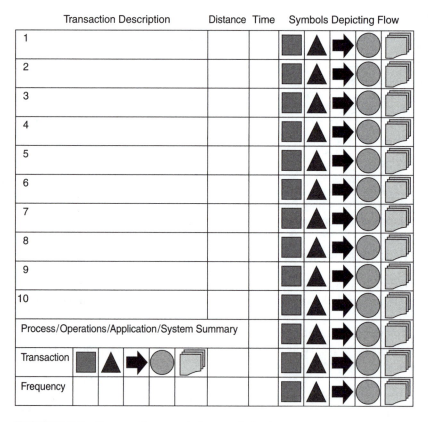

FIGURE 8.5   Process documentation worksheet.

for subsequent documentation in more formal flowcharts, frequently by using one of a variety of commercially available software packages.

HORIZONTAL FLOW PROCESS ANALYSIS

Horizontal flow process analysis is another specialized flowcharting technique used to simultaneously document interdepartmental, multiprocedural, and multi-personnel procedures.

Common examples include

- Supply requisition, purchase order creation, supply receipt, and distribution, charging, and patient billing
- Inpatient admission, transfers, and discharge
- Plant maintenance and operations work orders, response, and completion
- Laboratory and imaging requests in two dimensions depicting multifunctional responsibilities

This tool is most effective as an alternative to a lengthy narrative that would otherwise be necessary to describe complex processes, applications, or systems.

Figure 8.6 portrays this technique as each process is shown. This tool is also referred to as a deployment chart.

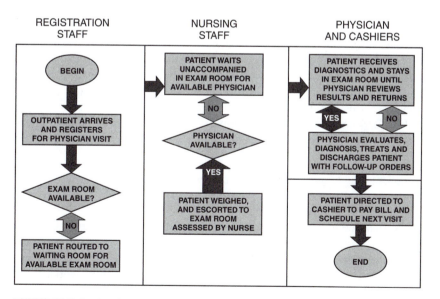

FIGURE 8.6 Horizontal or deployment flow chart: outpatient clinic process.

TIME FLOW ANALYSIS

This technique is used to qualify and quantify an individual's workday, to distribute workload more efficiently, to measure time lost to unpredictable and/or unproductive workload fluctuation, and to determine an activity's effectiveness. Time flow analysis is ideally suited for nonrepetitive, creative, and professional work.

Furthermore, time flow analysis identifies poorly planned work routines and/or extraneous duties detracting from efficient workflow. This technique is useful to substantiate personnel requests or position upgrades. Time flow analysis is a flexible tool used when well-defined tasks can be encoded to simplify data collection and analysis. Analysis is similar to that discussed for work distribution analysis, except that it can be much more accurate with significant worker involvement and cooperation.

Time increments in 2-minute activity segments over a 12-hour shift are a common presentation, as depicted in Figure 8.7. Spreadsheet workbooks make data collection easier and analysis more accurate and expeditious. Work simplification analysts must collaboratively develop a simple activity coding scheme to be used by staff to document each activity by code, sequence, and duration and by analysts to aggregate and analyze data collected. Some commercial products have fully automated this process by capturing activities with bar codes and generating real-time flow analysis.

JOB SEQUENCING

Job-sequencing techniques balance processing times among and between prioritized assignments. A primary objective of sequencing is to ensure that process components are configured with workstation idle time minimized while simultaneously maximizing throughput. These techniques reduce average turnaround time and increase operational efficiency.

Job-sequencing guidelines yield optimal scheduling and process improvement outcomes when detailed queuing theory, advanced analysis, and investment are unwarranted

- Select batch(es) with the shortest processing time first.
- A patient specimen batch is scheduled as early as possible when the shortest processing time is for the first workstation.
- A batch is scheduled as late as possible when the shortest processing time is for the second workstation.
- When batch processing times are identical at any workstation or there are already batches of shorter processing duration scheduled for a workstation, any subsequent batch scheduling may be random.
- As scheduled batches are eliminated from further consideration, sequencing and scheduling guidelines are repeated until all patient specimen batches are scheduled.

Employee Name	Position Title	Shift Start Time	Shift Start Time
_____	_____	_____	_____

TASK	TIME	TASK	TIME	TASK	TIME	TASK	TIME	TASK	TIME	TASK	TIME	TASK	TIME	TASK	TIME	TASK	TIME	TASK	TIME	TASK	TIME	TASK	TIME
0700		0800		0900		1000		1100		1200		0100		0200		0300		0400		0500		0600	
0702		0802		0902		1002		1102		1202		0102		0202		0302		0402		0502		0602	
0704		0804		0904		1004		1104		1204		0104		0204		0304		0404		0504		0604	
0706		0806		0906		1006		1106		1206		0106		0206		0306		0406		0506		0606	
0708		0808		0908		1008		1108		1208		0108		0208		0308		0408		0508		0608	
0710		0810		0910		1010		1110		1210		0110		0210		0310		0410		0510		0610	
0712		0812		0912		1012		1112		1212		0112		0212		0312		0412		0512		0612	
0714		0814		0914		1014		1114		1214		0114		0214		0314		0414		0514		0614	
0716		0816		0916		1016		1116		1216		0116		0216		0316		0416		0516		0616	
0718		0818		0918		1018		1118		1218		0118		0218		0318		0418		0518		0618	
0720		0820		0920		1020		1120		1220		0120		0220		0320		0420		0520		0620	
0722		0822		0922		1022		1122		1222		0122		0222		0322		0422		0522		0622	
0724		0824		0924		1024		1124		1224		0124		0224		0324		0424		0524		0624	
0726		0826		0926		1026		1126		1226		0126		0226		0326		0426		0526		0626	
0728		0828		0928		1028		1128		1228		0128		0228		0328		0428		0528		0628	
0730		0830		0930		1030		1130		1230		0130		0230		0330		0430		0530		0630	
0732		0832		0932		1032		1132		1232		0132		0232		0332		0432		0532		0632	
0734		0834		0934		1034		1134		1234		0134		0234		0334		0434		0534		0634	
0736		0836		0936		1036		1136		1236		0136		0236		0336		0436		0536		0636	
0738		0838		0938		1038		1138		1238		0138		0238		0338		0438		0538		0638	
0740		0840		0940		1040		1140		1240		0140		0240		0340		0440		0540		0640	
0742		0842		0942		1042		1142		1242		0142		0242		0342		0442		0542		0642	
0744		0844		0944		1044		1144		1244		0144		0244		0344		0444		0544		0644	
0746		0846		0946		1046		1146		1246		0146		0246		0346		0446		0546		0646	
0748		0848		0948		1048		1148		1248		0148		0248		0348		0448		0548		0648	
0750		0850		0950		1050		1150		1250		0150		0250		0350		0450		0550		0650	
0752		0852		0952		1052		1152		1252		0152		0252		0352		0752		0552		0652	
0754		0854		0954		1054		1154		1254		0154		0254		0354		0454		0554		0654	
0756		0856		0956		1056		1156		1256		0156		0256		0356		0456		0556		0656	
0758		0858		0958		1058		1158		1258		0158		0258		0358		0458		0558		0658	

Activity Codes:

A_____	E_____	I_____	M_____	Q_____	U_____
B_____	F_____	J_____	N_____	R_____	V_____
C_____	G_____	K_____	O_____	S_____	W_____
D_____	H_____	L_____	P_____	T_____	X_____

Supervisor Verification	Date
_____	_____

FIGURE 8.7   Time flow analysis data collection worksheet.

Using laboratory test processing as an example, a table is constructed to display expected processing times for each batch at each workstation.

Processes with shortest processing duration are completed first in highly stochastic environments with a high standard deviation of procedure times. These algorithms minimize mean flow time, procedure wait time, and procedure downtime. Each procedure is sequenced according to earliest required completion time. Although not always minimizing average wait time, maximum wait time is always minimized.

When scheduling multiple procedures to achieve high resource utilization, procedure sequencing should be based on shortest downtime or turnover time that a subsequent procedure can be started to minimize procedure, instrument, or other resource downtime.

More advanced job, task, and batch sequencing techniques are included in classic queuing theory.

Throughout any work simplification project, analysts are constantly questioning the level of detail to be included in any analysis. As a general rule, as more levels of detail are analyzed, more opportunities for improvement are likely to be identified. This rule should be applied judiciously. Otherwise, any work breakdown analysis risks becoming so bogged down in detail that obvious improvement opportunities get overlooked.

As illustrated to the right in Figure 8.8, this process of patient admission, diagnosis, treatment, and discharge could be studied at a relatively "high level" and would likely yield opportunities for improvement.

However, if each of these 4 tasks are broken down into more detail, that is, each task with 10 subtasks, 40 rather than 4 potential opportunities for process improvement become visible. This degree of depth is especially important in team efforts where experts of certain portions of a complex process are chartered as an improvement team and need to clearly understand an entire process, not just a portion within their area of responsibility.

Implications of these techniques illustrated by Figure 8.8 should be considered judiciously in conjunction with work breakdown analytic objectives.

As tactics outlined throughout this chapter coalesce, overall work breakdown strategy and obviously structured analytic approach to workflow and process analysis and improvement become obvious.

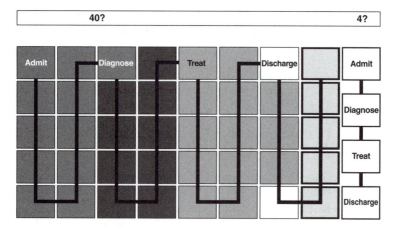

FIGURE 8.8   40 or 4 opportunities?

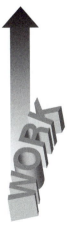

Workplace neat and orderly
Opposite, symmetric, balanced motions used
Rhythm smooth, natural and flowing motions
Keep motion path within normal work area

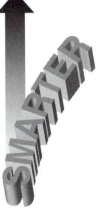

Smallest body member moving shortest distance
Materials prepositioned for worker by power or gravity
Avoid unnecessary motions
Remove idleness from motion path
Tools prepositioned and ready for use
Employ aids, clamps, and guides for repetitive work
Relieve hands by foot controls, chutes, and drop delivery

FIGURE 8.9 Working smarter, not harder.

125

SUMMARY

This chapter reviewed classic work simplification techniques: work distribution, flow process, time flow analysis, horizontal flow process analysis, deployment flow, and job sequencing.

Basic concepts and the classic eight steps of process improvement were discussed.

In addition, the traditional industrial engineering methodology, symbolized by the mnemonic "Work Smarter" (Figure 8.9), was presented.

Fundamental concepts included

- Work distribution
- Why techniques
- Work simplification objects and approaches
- Flow process analysis and documentation
- Time flow analysis
- Job sequencing

CHAPTER QUESTIONS

These questions reinforce student understanding, learning, and retention while stimulating class discussion:

1. What is work distribution?
2. Explain the why technique.
3. How is time flow analysis used?

ADDITIONAL RESOURCES

These references are recommended for additional reading and more comprehensive content beyond the scope of this book.

Griffith, J., White, K. (2002). The Well-Managed Healthcare Organization. Chicago: Health Administration Press.

Larson, J. (2001). Management Engineering. Chicago: Healthcare Information and Management Systems Society.

Seidel, L., Gorsky, R., Lewis, J. (1995). Applied Quantitative Methods for Health Services Management. Baltimore, MD: Health Professions Press.

Veney, J., Kaluzny, A. (1998). Evaluation and Decision Making for Health Services. Chicago: Health Administration Press.

Wan, T. (1995). Analysis and Evaluation of Health Care Systems: An Integrated Approach to Managerial Decision Making. Baltimore, MD: Health Professions Press.

CHAPTER 9

Tactical Performance Management and Metrics: Productivity Benchmarking for Operations Improvement

This chapter introduces performance management using productivity measurement and labor resource benchmarks that focus on these concepts:

- Productivity definitions and fundamental metrics
- Scheduling, monitoring, and improving labor utilization
- Labor resource management tools and techniques
- Staffing benchmarks and productivity indexing

An understanding of the definition of productivity and an appreciation of the variability of underlying qualifiers and assumptions are necessary because these definitions are very venue specific and increasingly quantitative in nature.

Productivity is defined with subtle differences within each healthcare venue and is very dependent on context and varying perspectives (nurses and other clinical professionals, health economists, hospital administrators, management engineers, systems analysts).

Classic definitions of productivity with examples of their context are as follows:

- A ratio of outputs to inputs; Conversely, inputs required to produce a unit of output
- Generically, a relationship between inputs and outputs
- Quantity and quality of output produced by a fixed amount of input where input reflects available hours
- Ratio of services required to hours expended
- Ratio of services required to hours expended with an adjustment for quality
- Ratio of work output to work input
- Relationship between acceptable output and required input necessary to achieve a desired outcome
- Ratio of required care or service intensity to equivalent available hours, adjusted by an expression of quality
- Value added during patient access, diagnosis, treatment, education, rehabilitation, and follow-up (sum of process inputs required for patient outcome)
- Ratio of output to input, where output is represented by DRG-based patient care reimbursement received for inpatient care and services provided

Figure 9.1 expresses productivity as straightforward percentages in an arithmetic format. These expressions reflect an underlying principle that any valid productivity increase is based on any and all of the four options depicted in Figure 9.2. Therefore increasing productive healthcare delivery in any venue is only possible by making a change to a process that results in any of these fundamental options. Although often expressed in more complex or very descriptive terms in any unique situation, realistically only a single option, a combination, or a permutation of these relationships is valid.

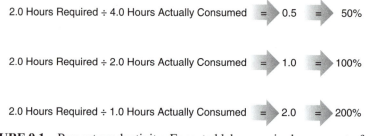

FIGURE 9.1   Percent productivity: Expected labor required as percent of actual labor resource consumed.

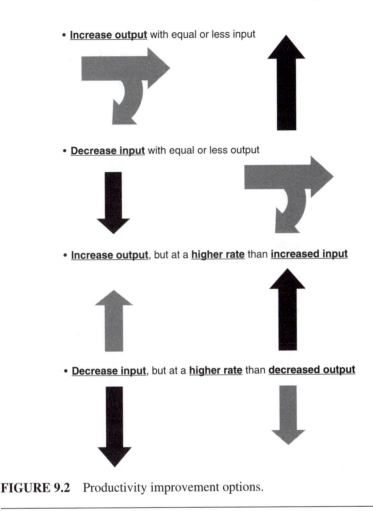

FIGURE 9.2   Productivity improvement options.

PRODUCTIVITY METRICS

Each unique productivity ratio (labor standard) is engineered in conjunction with variable units of measure that are relevant in each department or operational unit. These units of measure are determined from a variety of different sources and are ideally derived in real time from process data. These sources are discussed in detail throughout this and other chapters and are usually compared with standardized industrial benchmarks or uniquely engineered standards developed for operational units with very unique or nonstandard procedures. Over time a number of professional discipline-specific organizations led these benchmarking initiatives. The

American Society of Clinical Pathologists and the Chicago Hospital Council pioneered the development of procedure-specific standardized databases of "workload units." Workload, staffing, and productivity metrics, have provided annual updates for more than 20 years. These standardized units of measure are linked with an appropriate volume indicator that represents key departmental functions. For example, nursing units of measure are almost always patient days (a count of patients receiving care each day). Emergency departments track patient visits, whereas laboratories use billed laboratory tests as workload units, or units of measure.

These common underlying qualifiers or frequently encountered assumptions are represented by numerical expressions that must be mastered to understand productivity metrics and related concepts:

- *Costs and related productivity* address direct care or service costs as well as supervision, management and support staffing, in-service education mandates, administration, and other overhead costs.
- *Direct care or service costs* must address key aspects of "hands-on" patient care, diagnostic, therapeutic, or nursing costs necessary to incorporate all resource requirements, infrastructure, and related expenses necessary for well-managed patient care delivery.
- *Indirect care or service costs* must address all other resources and costs. For example, recruitment, orientation, overtime, on-call pay, shift differential, and in-service education programs are allocated proportionally to all patients, even if individual patients did not receive any direct benefit.

Indirect and other allocated labor-related costs for paid time off (vacation, sick days, holidays, employee benefits, etc.) must be addressed. Usually, these costs reflect an additional 35% to 45% burden to an employee's paid wage rate. For example, an employee paid at $20.00 per hour worked reflects an additional cost of $8.00 to $10.00 paid per hour worked, adjusting for non-productive time of 12% to 15% for benefits such as vacation, sick, and holiday pay. Another 25% to 30% expense is associated with employer-paid costs such as pension, social security contributions, workers' compensation, unemployment insurance health care, and other benefit costs. As a result of these additional burdens, an employee paid $20.00 an hour costs a provider $28.00 to $30.00 for each care hour delivered.

LABOR COSTS AND BENCHMARKS

Productive hours can be further disaggregated into fixed and variable components because some positions fluctuate with workload volume. This category includes nurses, respiratory therapists, radiology technologists, and others directly involved in delivery of units of measure for each department. Managers and unit secretaries are typically classified as fixed positions. These positions usually support direct caregiver performance. Some organizations separate fixed positions into direct and indirect positions.

Direct fixed time accounts for time involved in direct support of operations (a manager or unit secretary). Indirect fixed time may be time used to prepare or to plan for change, such as employee orientation, education, training, and staff meetings. Historically, most organizations do not plan at this level of detail, but as upgrades to legacy information systems enable such analysis, each process is better understood. Theoretically, any employee can be assigned to perform any required task with appropriate training. This postulation implies that managers throughout an organization have a high level of control over productive hours and costs. Alternatively, managers have much less control over nonproductive hours (vacation, sick leave, etc.) and related costs.

Historically, organizations only use labor hours expended as an input variable in productivity calculations. With the advent of managed care as well as dramatic and volatile increases in the cost of care, paid hours or dollars per unit of measure evolved as primary indicators. These metrics are used together, enabling managers to better understand and more effectively manage increasingly scarce, expensive labor and other resources.

Traditionally, management engineers have been recognized as healthcare provider organizations' productivity "subject matter" experts in facilities of sufficient size and resources to justify these internal staff positions. Alternatively, these specialized "management science and operations research" professional services are provided by management engineering staff from consulting firms who are contracted as needed. Core productivity concepts have not changed materially over time, but continual refinement of benchmarks, metrics, analytic technology, and reporting formats has been ongoing. Traditional industrial engineering techniques developed in manufacturing settings in the early years of the 20th century have been introduced and emulated in various service industries, including health care, in the last quarter century.

This evolutionary process occurred simultaneously within disciplinary, organizational, healthcare operations research, and systems development "silos." Initial productivity metrics were developed and refined in hospitals because large concentrations of labor and cost consumption demanded increasingly robust management and monitoring tools and techniques to manage organizational performance. Productivity measures necessarily changed as hospitals grew and evolved into complex and diverse healthcare delivery systems (clinics, extended care facilities, home health agencies, physician offices, diagnostic centers, rehabilitation facilities, ambulatory surgical centers, and health plans).

Mastering these concepts is an essential competency of healthcare professionals participating in systems design, development, implementation, or operations as well as in quality management; continuous process improvement; administrative, clinical, or support operations; operations analysis; and management engineering. These professionals must be proficient with these metrics and underlying operational analytics. Together with work measurement, work simplification, operations analysis, process improvement, and staffing analysis, these productivity benchmarking concepts are required to effectively, efficiently, and safely manage skilled, scarce, and expensive resources necessary to provide quality health care in virtually any delivery venue.

Table 9.1 highlights units of measure and related contemporary labor standards expressed in terms of paid time per unit of measure. Historically, productivity and resource management techniques and benchmark standardization in individual departments used a relative value unit as a standard unit of measure. This traditional practice was common until more rigorous analysis produced credible, increasingly more quantitative and precise labor standards.

TABLE 9.1   Example of Labor Standards per Unit of Measure by Department

Representative Departments	Unit of Measure	Paid Hours Per Unit
Nursing		
Intensive Care	Acuity-Adjusted Patient Days	20
Medical and Surgical	Acuity-Adjusted Patient Days	7
Newborn Nursery	Acuity-Adjusted Patient Days	4
Obstetrics/Gynecology	Acuity-Adjusted Patient Days	8
Pediatrics	Acuity-Adjusted Patient Days	7
Others		
Surgical Suite	Billed cases	12–15
Emergency Services	Billed visits	2–3
Outpatient Clinics	Billed visits	1–2
Laboratory Services	Billed tests	0.3–0.4
Diagnostic Imaging	Billed procedures	1–2
Human Resources	Full-time equivalent employees	13–16
Registration/Patient Accounting	Patient registrations	0.5–1.0

All units of measure benchmarks as hours per unit of measure are for illustration only. Provider specific values are proprietary.

A relative value unit reflects a weighted volume unit, occasionally used in ancillary and other departments where traditional volume varies dramatically in terms of length, complexity, or intensity. For example, a unit of measure in a radiology department may reflect a composite of a number of unique procedures. Each procedure is by definition not the same as another. For example, a simple chest or ankle x-ray may require 15 minutes to complete and a diagnostic angiography procedure may require 60 or more minutes to complete.

A relative value unit algorithm approximates cumulative workload requirements in a department or organizational unit with a weighting multiplier for each procedure's workload labor standard (unit of measure and volume of each procedure performed). Since most acute care was historically provided in inpatient venues, many units of measure incorporated key operations-wide statistics (admissions, discharges, patient days, and occupied beds) that were adjusted for average patient acuity. Because more acute care is increasingly completed in an outpatient setting rather than as an inpatient (more than 70% of surgical cases are provided on an outpatient basis), use of these "adjusted" units of measure have decreased and unique units of measure (workload or labor standards) have been developed in other healthcare venues in addition to inpatient acute care hospitals.

As providers reorganize, reengineer, and refine processes and staffing patterns, incorporating department-specific "skill mix" requirements, fewer highly paid but underused employees are hired, resulting in fewer paid hours per unit of measure. For example, fewer registered nurses may be assigned to a nursing unit and more licensed practical nurses added at lower wage rates. Such an organizational change may result in a lower cost per unit of measure. When assessed from both a professional challenge and financial perspective, this change is likely positive.

Positive quality and operational performance may be also achieved when fewer higher paid staff improve a department's hours per unit of measure but have a negative impact on cost per unit of measure. Most progressive organizations track both indicators, usually considering the cost per unit of measure first. In many cases these changes are implemented because of a variety of both internal and external environmental factors, such as staffing shortages.

Having highlighted traditional aspects of productivity development and ongoing refinements since the early 1960s, the rest of this chapter focuses on contemporary productivity data and derived information to more tactically manage labor resources to increase performance per paid hour to improve healthcare delivery effectiveness. More fundamentally, operational elements of these tools are used as productivity drivers and metrics to track operational performance improvement and digital transformation. These are resource management concepts that aspiring systems analysts and operations research professionals must demonstrate competency to understand, explain, train, and redesign processes and systems.

These resource management tools and techniques enable operations managers to assess departmental and overall organization performance:

- Productivity indexing
- Workforce planning
- Resource allocation
- Control of labor expenses and budgeting
- Benchmarking

PRODUCTIVITY INDEXING

A productivity index is calculated to "normalize" departmental standard reporting in a credible manner to enhance both manager and senior leadership confidence in the utility of these tools. By ensuring that "apples-to-apples" comparisons are equitable, these techniques are used by managers to longitudinally evaluate performance trends, as well as department operating effectiveness.

BENCHMARKING

Target values are determined with many different approaches, such as detailed staffing/operations analysis, historical performance ratios, external benchmarking comparisons or laboring relations negotiation. A productivity index or percentage of productivity is reported to comparatively track productivity in each department relative to others within an organization or IDS. Unique productivity metrics are used to ensure that accurate reporting of labor standards is developed to be meaningful to department managers. Although productivity can be accurately determined within a department, comparative department performance reporting throughout an organization must be indexed to be equitable.

WORKFORCE PLANNING AND RESOURCE ALLOCATION

Actual productivity performance and labor expense per unit of measure, are compared for a specified period with each department's unique target ratios. For example, a productivity index greater than 100% indicates that actual performance is greater than the standard or targeted performance expectations for this department. Alternatively, when a productivity index for a department is less than 100%, departmental performance is less than targeted performance also shown in Figure 9.1.

Realistic productivity performance indices usually fluctuate within a range of 95% to 105%. Establishing these expectations requires a series of productivity studies to refine reporting data so that both department management and staff trust this component of performance reporting as do senior managers.

When a target value equals maximum capacity of current departmental processes and systems, the productivity index is expressed as 100%. Managers become more creative with staffing assignments and allocation of resources as they gain confidence and collaborate with peers to challenge and ultimately validate the credibility of accurate productivity reporting.

Experience often demonstrates that process and productivity problems are systemic in nature and are not employee initiated. Put another way, analysts often discover that "good people" are trying their best but are frustrated by poor systems. Specifically, by objectively determining how long it takes to perform a specific procedure, treatment, process, or service, realistic performance expectations are established and fairly used.

For example, if the standard time to complete a chest x-ray is 15 minutes, with an additional 10 minutes for each patient to finish an initial check-in process, radiology department receptionists can advise patients to expect to be in the department for 25 minutes. Providing this type of information to patients treated on an outpatient basis is very important, because they may have made plans to be available for a limited amount of time. Obviously, not all services have such definite duration, but for those that do productivity information can help manage patient expectations.

RESOURCE SCHEDULING

Effective scheduling requires continual refining of processes and procedures that are beneficial to both providers and patients by increasing patient convenience and by reducing each patient's length of stay. Productivity information is best used to determine short-term scheduling, long-term staffing, and workforce needs. Strategically, important long-term workforce planning defines expected labor costs from required hour ratios per unit of measure, current skill mix, and projected workload volume.

By applying "what if" scenarios or precise process simulation of personnel availability or optimal skill mix, an operations analyst can predict future workforce needs. By performing a "gap analysis" that compares future to current state, a strategic plan can be developed to address identified deficits.

CONTROL OF LABOR EXPENSES AND BUDGETING

Labor and labor-related benefit costs exceed 60% of total operations expenses for most healthcare providers. "You cannot manage what you do not measure" is an old adage that is very appropriate in this circumstance because these scarce, skilled, and expensive resources must be continually measured and monitored to ultimately be effectively managed.

Productivity management training, protocols and systems enable first-line supervisors, department managers, and senior leaders to skillfully measure, manage, and control these mission critical resources and associated costs. Organizational benefits to be realized from these investments include

- *Understanding* true labor costs to enable management at all organizational levels to identify areas for improvement or cost reduction
- *Identifying* increasing cost trends, either within a single department or throughout an organization
- *Developing* proactive plans of action to eliminate or slow undesired increases
- *Implementing* realistic action plans, leading to reduced costs and an improved organization bottom line

Use of a well-designed productivity management system facilitates appropriate resource allocation. Annual budget processes require each department to demonstrate effective use of assigned resources in the previous year and to credibly justify any requests for departmental position increases.

A well-designed and effectively functioning productivity management system enables senior management to allocate resources to those departments with demonstrated need and to reassign resources from areas that have not demonstrated need. When periodic workforce shortages occur, management has an ability to objectively assign and reassign resources to those "high priority" areas demonstrating most critical needs.

Appropriate staffing assignments can be made when labor requirements for specific workload at specified patient acuity and service demands are understood. Staffing needs within health care are quite volatile, as are periodic shortages of appropriately trained and available workers.

Understanding fundamental productivity management principles is a sound foundation for healthcare organizations as is investing in workforce planning and forecasting to determine the required number of personnel by skill type. Without credible productivity management systems, department managers and senior leaders find this process very difficult, if not impossible. Increasing healthcare costs are continuing to challenge providers to streamline operations by continuous process improvement and BPR, because even leaner budgets are inevitable. Installing and maintaining an effective productivity management system is a prudent, proactive countermeasure. An upward-spiraling cycle of more effective operations results from well-managed workforce productivity. These improvements engender budgets that result in better managed productivity, which produces even better budgets, and so on. Ultimately, these operations management improvements produce a higher performing organization. Productivity monitoring and management are conceptually simple yet powerful tools to realize improvement opportunities. These opportunities further enable organizations to better use skilled, scarce, and increasingly expensive labor resources.

Many third-party productivity systems are available from commercial vendors such as Solucient, Premier, and Data Advantage for purchase, lease, or license. Firms such as Applied Management Systems, Barrick & Associates, and other larger consulting, accounting, and auditing firms provide in-depth consulting support and competitive benchmarks to assist providers to understand these metrics, implement operational or management changes, and improve organizational performance.

OUTCOMES

Many organizations have developed internal systems using database or spreadsheet programs. These systems differ in a variety of ways. For example:

- Credibility
- Sophistication
- Detail display and maintenance
- Reporting capabilities (graphs, multiple period reporting, etc.)

Often, large healthcare providers and health plans develop internal and external productivity monitoring and performance management systems. These systems or applications report shift-by-shift, daily, weekly, biweekly, monthly, quarterly, or annual metrics to measure organizational performance compared to variable historical reporting period performance.

Comparing departments or divisions against themselves over time is useful to identify and track significant trends. This technique may be used alone or in conjunction with other performance metrics. Typically, department managers and division directors view these data and comparative metrics with more credibility. Information produced using these productivity metrics often provide data and information used to develop future budgets, and identify ongoing process improvement. Other operations research tools discussed in this text (work simplification and operations analysis or more advanced topics such as process simulation) are used to establish credible baseline performance.

Staffing analyses are a direct result of applying productivity information to specific processes or departments. A thorough understanding of how and why productivity systems work is necessary for systems analysts and management engineers because these disciplines are usually involved in promoting expected process improvements.

SUMMARY

This chapter introduced and discussed measurement and terminology, tools, techniques, and concepts to understand how productivity measurement and performance management are essential to effective and efficient delivery of patient care. Simply and generically defined, productivity is a ratio of outputs to inputs or, conversely, of inputs required to produce a unit of output.

Fundamental concepts and content focused on

- Productivity definitions and fundamental metrics
- Scheduling, monitoring, and improving labor utilization
- Labor resource management tools and techniques
- Staffing benchmarks and productivity indexing

CHAPTER QUESTIONS

These questions reinforce student understanding, learning, and retention while stimulating class discussion:

1. List three common definitions of productivity and examples of context in which each is used.
2. Explain the difference between productivity and target utilization indexing from the perspective of a department manager and a chief executive officer in a healthcare organization.
3. Describe the expected range of productivity percentages in an appropriately staffed department that meets quality and performance expectations in a provider organization.
4. Show example calculations for 80%, 100%, and 120% productivity and explain in simple terms four ways to improve each.

ADDITIONAL RESOURCES

These references are recommended for additional reading and more comprehensive content beyond the scope of this book.

Griffith, J., White, K. (2002). The Well-Managed Healthcare Organization. Chicago: Health Administration Press.

Larson, J. (2001). Management Engineering. Chicago: Healthcare Information and Management Systems Society.

Longest, Jr., B., Rakich, J., Darr, K. (2004). Managing Health Services Organizations and Systems. Baltimore, MD: Health Professions Press.

Seidel, L., Gorsky, R., Lewis, J. (1995). Applied Quantitative Methods for Health Services Management. Baltimore, MD: Health Professions Press.

Veney, J., Kaluzny, A. (1998). Evaluation and Decision Making for Health Services. Chicago: Health Administration Press.

Wan, T. (1995). Analysis and Evaluation of Health Care Systems: An Integrated Approach to Managerial Decision Making. Baltimore, MD: Health Professions Press.

CHAPTER 10

Queuing Theory and Waiting Line Analysis

This chapter introduces queuing theory or waiting line analysis, focusing on:

- Queuing applications throughout healthcare provider organizations
- Line balancing by tolerable waiting versus provider productivity
- Poisson arrival distribution probability
- Exponential service distribution probability
- Balancing idle provider time and patient waiting time

Queuing, or waiting line analysis, is a set of equations that calculate waiting time, line length, and other parameters from average patient volume, service time, and staffing levels.

Key queuing objectives are

- Data collection, aggregation, and analysis of arrival rates
- Proficiency in management and control of jockeying and reneging rates, balking, batching, and "first in, first out processing"
- Productive and quality service delivery without unacceptable resource idle time
- Waiting line management resulting in effective and efficient use of resources that are delicately balanced with patient expectations of minimal waiting time and high quality service

These challenging objectives are achieved with optimal resource utilization at acceptable cost. Queuing service models and analysts achieve increased demands for prompt service weighed against minimal or no waiting (no line or acceptably short lines) without unacceptable server idle time. Queuing analysis, frequently using computer simulation models, is a technique that identifies and analyzes process bottlenecks and assesses various options to cost-effectively improve processing components while reducing patient waiting and server idle time to improve productivity and reduce service delivery cost.

WAITING LINE BALANCING

Most patients find waiting lines, especially waiting lines that are too long, to be an irritating but unavoidable factor of contemporary healthcare delivery. Patients, especially those who are seriously ill, cannot, will not, or do not like to wait. From an outpatient's perspective, waiting is idle and nonproductive time and may result in lost wages. From a service provider's perspective, a line represents demand for service. From a manager's perspective, waiting line management is a challenge requiring a dynamic balance between patient sensitivity and a cost-effective service delivery.

Common examples of queuing applications in healthcare delivery include

- Patients waiting for service
- Laboratory specimens waiting for processing, analysis, and result reporting
- Patient accounts waiting for third-party reimbursement and patient billing
- Physician orders awaiting timely fulfillment and follow-up
- Prescriptions waiting to be filled
- Images waiting for radiologist interpretation

Effective application of information technology will digitally transform these aspects of care delivery with dramatic improvements in process efficiency, provider performance, and organizational effectiveness. These improvements fundamentally alter patient perspectives, reduce costs, and significantly increase patient satisfaction.

Anyone or anything waiting in a line is considered a patient. Service provided to each patient is referred to as a unit of service, and each staff member providing a unit of service is referred to as a server. Most healthcare processes are complex and therefore reflect multiple services provided by multiple servers. Complex concepts beyond single-server queues are beyond the scope of this book.

As long as a line of patients is present, each server has an opportunity to engage in productive activity (serving each patient, resident, or client). When no line exists each server is idle. Idle servers are not productive components of healthcare delivery systems. Requiring patients to wait in a line for service ensures that a server is productive. If no patient is in line, a server is considered to be idle and unproductively waiting for another patient to enter a queue.

Frequently patients, residents, or clients are not actually present in a queue but are represented as specimens, documents, and so on. These specimens and documents are just as critical to prompt and effective care delivery as patients, residents, or clients themselves and must be perceived as such.

Providing a service requires and consumes resources. For example, filling a prescription requires pharmacist time and supplies necessary to fulfill the demand represented by each prescription. The length of time a patient waits in a line for the prescription to be filled depends on the number of pharmacists on duty to fill prescriptions, as well as any pharmacist's time required to fill prescriptions for those patients who arrived earlier. Theoretically, the time a patient waits in a queue can be reduced by adding additional pharmacists and/or other resources (pharmacy technicians). If demand fluctuates and too many pharmacists or pharmacy technicians are added, some servers will be idle and not necessarily engaged in productive activity.

In an ambulatory care clinic one physician, nurse, technologist, or therapist may evaluate and treat at least three patients per hour. At this rate if one additional clinician (server) is added, six patients rather than three would be treated each hour.

As resources are added to a service process (adding an additional clinician *or* support staff member), service speed or processing rate increases the number of patients simultaneously evaluated and treated in this process. However from a practical perspective, service process or provider systems have a finite capacity to deliver patient service because of a limitation on service space or available examination rooms.

Another example: a facility with three surgical suites can only simultaneously perform three surgeries. If surgery demand is greater than three patients at one time, some patients must wait. A computed tomography (CT) scanner may be technically capable of processing 100 scans per hour, regardless of available staffing supporting the scanner.

From a strategic planning perspective, bed need determinations in most state health departments require a certificate of need (CON) to justify licensing of additional hospital or nursing home beds in a geographically defined service area use. An 85% occupancy rate for existing beds is a common prerequisite to any further consideration. Actual bed need determination on a regional or state-wide level is determined by using queuing theory, with "occupied beds" as service units and "average length of stay" (ALOS) as service time. Few new beds were licensed during the last decade because lengths of stay were dramatically reduced as managed care limited reimbursement per stay. More recently, after hospital lengths of stay stabilized and demographic demand increased, additional beds are considered necessary to provide timely access to inpatient hospital or nursing home care.

Legacy healthcare delivery processes or systems were designed with an average productivity of 80%, with a surge capacity of potentially 90%. Indirect care delivery time of 20% is then expected to be devoted to other non-service activities, such as documentation, preventive maintenance, and stocking supplies.

Provider managers face dual and frequently conflicting conundrums as they are increasingly challenged to balance patient waiting times with resources consumed to provide quality, timely, and cost-effective care. Idle staff, equipment, and other costly resources such as surgical suites do not benefit hospitals or physicians and may risk financial viability of both parties. Patient-sensitive healthcare administrators expect personnel and medical staff to provide quality services as needed, recognizing that a patient should not wait for surgery or treatment, because any delay in providing a service is rarely, if ever therapeutic.

Long delays lead to deterioration in a patient's condition or in processing a laboratory specimen awaiting analysis. Although short delays are sometimes acceptable from a clinical perspective, a definition of what constitutes a long or short delay usually depends on unique and situation-specific circumstances. Twenty minutes may constitute too much delay for a medical test or procedure, depending on a patient's condition. However, 10 minutes may be a short delay for a patient to be seen by a physician in ambulatory care. Clinical acceptability or unacceptability of delay in any process providing service varies based on clinical and medical considerations.

A patient's acceptance of a delay also may affect patient participation in current or future services. From a strategic perspective, savvy administrators strive to build and sustain effective organizational processes with efficient service delivery systems and subsystems. At a more tactical level, managers are expected to balance acceptable waiting times with optimal use of scarce expensive resources necessary to provide these services.

This delicate balancing act is expected of competent managers throughout service delivery systems. In some instances service systems are managed by advising patients (units) when to arrive. For example, most physicians in private practice schedule patient appointments to ensure optimal physician efficiency within the limits of a patient's tolerance for unacceptably long queues. Frequently, physician schedules are "double booked" to meet extraordinary demand. Most non-emergent patient admissions to a hospital are scheduled by providing an appointment at a given day and time. Surgeons are scheduled to use a specified start time or block in an operating room in the surgical suite of the hospital or an outpatient surgical center.

Staff are scheduled to minimize any patient or physician waiting for service delivery by maintaining a constant demand, that is, leveling of workload over time for a service that can be met with existing resources. For other more urgent situations, special procedures are used to manage service systems; for example a physician can order a "stat" procedure, which comes from the Latin *statim*, meaning "at once" or "immediately."

For example, a patient's blood specimen is rushed to the clinical laboratory and processed ahead of any other tests to provide prompt results to a physician. In hospital emergency rooms patients are seen and evaluated and then placed in a service queue based on medical need, not the order in which they arrived for service. This type of service system is referred to as medical triaging or "fast tracking." Thus in a hospital emergency room a patient may remain last in line as long as patients with more acute needs arrive and demand service with more urgent service requirements. Sequencing or ordering of patients in queues is continually reevaluated every time another patient arrives based on each patient's medical need.

> Random arrivals are unscheduled arrivals not influenced by previous patient arrivals or departures.

Random arrival means that probability governs arrivals within specified time periods. For example, if an average of six patients arrives in an hour, this does not mean that every patient arrives exactly 10 minutes apart. Some probability exists that all patients will arrive at one time, just as there is a probability that each patient will arrive every 10 minutes during a 1-hour period of time. First in, first out (FIFO) means that service delivery order is determined by patient arrival sequence.

SINGLE CHANNEL, SINGLE SERVER

Servers are channels (professionals, paraprofessionals, and administrative and support staff) providing service to patients. The number of channels reflect the number of servers available to arriving patients. Some service delivery systems are designed to have a single channel of servers, whereas other systems are designed with multiple channels. For example, supermarkets use many cashiers in checkout stations, whereas banks and airline reservation counters use one line to feed multiple servers (tellers and reservation agents) in multiple-channel systems.

Following are key terms and concepts associated with queuing or waiting line analysis and the context in which used:

- *Balking* occurs when a patient, upon discovering an unacceptable length of a line, refuses to enter the queue.
- *Reneging* occurs as a patient waits in line for awhile, deciding that this wait is unacceptable and leaves the queue.

- *Batching* occurs when groups of patients can be served simultaneously (e.g., expectant parents receiving prenatal education in a classroom with other couples).
- *Jockeying* occurs as a patient chooses one queue but then decides that another queue is shorter and changes lines.

PROBABILITY DISTRIBUTIONS

Poisson probability distributions are used to estimate patterns in which patients arrive for service. Poisson distributions are considered more appropriate estimates of random arrival patterns than a "normal probability" distribution. Unlike a normal probability distribution that is symmetric and bell shaped, a Poisson distribution has a long tail and by definition is not symmetric.

A normal distribution assigns equal probabilities to values on either side of a mean, whereas a Poisson distribution recognizes that random arrival rates cluster about a mean, cannot be less than zero, and have a low probability of being much higher than the mean. In more complex situations, a Poisson probability distribution may not capture arrival and service time patterns. When this occurs more sophisticated probability distributions are used for waiting line model development. To simplify discussion, queuing theory models presented in this chapter are based on Poisson distributions to estimate random arrival patterns, thereby recognizing that these applications and issues are reserved for more advanced study.

Throughout this chapter these assumptions apply:

- Poisson probability distribution of arrivals is considered appropriate.
- Exponential probability distribution of service times is considered appropriate.
- Lines to be analyzed are governed by FIFO.
- No balking, reneging, or jockeying occurs.
- No services are batched.
- Patient populations to be served are infinite.

Using these assumptions, queuing models accurately simulate waiting based on the number of channels (lines) and the number of servers. For example,

- As arrival rates approach service rates, a waiting line will get longer as processing idle time decreases.
- When arrival rates are less than service rates, waiting lines will be shorter and processing idle time will increase.
- If an arrival rate is significantly greater than a related service rate, waiting lines will increase exponentially, theoretically approaching infinity.

Using these simplifying criteria, systems must be designed with a service rate greater than expected arrival rates. Queuing theory is an excellent concept with straightforward tools and techniques to understand, manage, modify and explain waiting line behavior *only* when service rates are higher than arrival rates.

This chapter limits further technical and theoretical discussion to only single-server single-line models, that are common in many healthcare delivery venues.

A variety of commercial analytic modeling software is available to build models. These models enable managers to simulate and dynamically analyze service demands by balancing system capacity to provide optimal patient service with only acceptable waiting for service. A service time probability distribution estimates time required to provide a unit of service. Unlike a normal data distribution, an exponential probability distribution suggests that service times will be greater than zero and more frequently short than long. Analytical models such as these can be used to analyze any linear or nonlinear operation to support and justify decision-making about patient waiting, provider productivity, lines, and service systems. More complex models of this type are addressed in Chapter 11, which focuses on simulation tools and techniques.

> Queuing theory uses an exponential probability distribution to describe service times. Using Poisson probability distributions of arrival times and exponential probability distributions of service times in tandem are appropriate for elementary modeling and analyzing waiting lines.

If a Poisson probability distribution and/or an exponential probability distribution are found to be inappropriate, other models and approaches must be used. Computer simulation is commonly used to develop and analyze an appropriate probability distribution to best model desired circumstances.

A single channel single-server system has one server and one line with these characteristics:

- Probability that service facility is idle
- Average number of patients in process
- Average time a patient spends in process, including both waiting and service time
- Average number of patients in queue waiting for service

An unbalanced single channel single-server system implies an idle system and an idle server (no patients are experiencing any wait for service); whereas a busy system means a patient must wait for service.

EXPONENTIAL PROBABILITY DISTRIBUTIONS

Calculations, observations, and analysis are necessary to highlight a Poisson and an exponential probability distribution that realistically presents options and trade-offs for management consideration. Actual decision-making is the prerogative and role of management, *not* an analytical model, tool, or technique. Ideally, a model is informative and useful in identifying and clarifying realistic options, alternatives, and implications.

Queuing theory incorporates these data distributions and specific equations to determine:

- Percentage of time that a server or service facility is idle
- Probability of a specific number of patients in service process
- Average number of patients in process
- Average time each patient spends waiting and served in process
- Average number of patients in a queue
- Average time that each patient is in a queue
- Percentage of time that an arriving patient must wait for service
- Probability that an arriving patient must wait for service

When considered with additional information (service costs, patient waiting limitations, space availability, equipment capacity, etc.), this information provides systems analysts, operations analysts, management engineers, and operations managers with ample information to analyze, design, and iteratively redesign waiting lines. Queuing theory is used in both systems development and ongoing operations analysis, enabling analysts, engineers, and operations management. These techniques provide in-depth insight into processes by examining interactions of these variable system capabilities, application components, and differing environmental considerations.

Processes bottlenecks can be easily studied. Options and applications can be identified and evaluated through analyses of these key statistics, such as arrival times, process length, and service departure times. For example, in a walk-in ambulatory care clinic a simple system to be studied by using queuing theory may include a patient waiting room and examination rooms used by nurses and physicians to diagnose and treat patients.

Waiting line analytic tools and queuing theory concepts are the most widely used and most effective operations research techniques to manage relationships between and among patients.and resources required to provide patient-centric, digitally transformed, and efficient care delivery in virtually any service setting. In addition to those applications mentioned earlier, patient appointment and surgical scheduling, capacity planning for acute care hospital bed requirements, examination room utilization, physician and surgical staff productivity are other common examples of queuing theory applications in health care.

Senior leadership support is required to sustain ongoing system operations and maintenance using exponential probability distribution of service times and queuing lines with both single-line and multichannel processes. Analytical systems must support Poisson probability distribution analyses of patient arrivals and throughput processing. "High-end" operations and production systems include queuing applications that derive required statistics from actual operations and are network based, having been designed to feed commercially available process—models and simulation applications in a real-world environment on a real-time basis. Queuing tools and techniques require knowledge, understanding, and proficiency in model design and implementation. Queuing analysts using these tools to study systems and processes must demonstrate technical and analytic proficiency.

SUMMARY

This chapter introduced and explained terminology, tools, techniques, and concepts in sufficient detail for a student to understand and learn queuing theory and waiting line analysis. Complex situations, examples, or calculations were excluded to facilitate mastery of essential concepts that are further explained with simulation and modeling applications.

Fundamental concepts and content highlighted were

- Applications throughout healthcare provider organizations
- Line-balancing of tolerable waiting versus provider productivity
- Poisson arrival distribution probability
- Exponential service distribution probability
- Balancing idle provider time and patient waiting time

CHAPTER QUESTIONS

These questions reinforce student understanding, learning, and retention while stimulating class discussion:

1. Identify and explain three common circumstances where queuing theory and waiting line analysis would be appropriate tools to facilitate the digital transformation of processes. Do *not* use examples described in this chapter.
2. What are balking, reneging, batching, and jockeying and how is each applicable to Poisson distribution-based queuing theory?
3. Describe how average, probability, and percentage calculations are related to waiting line analysis and their use in reporting results of a queuing analysis. Include examples that were *not* identified in this chapter.

4. How do arrival rates and service times interact and what happens if one or both are increased or decreased?
5. Briefly summarize key characteristics of a single-channel single-server model.
6. What are four examples of additional operational information that an administrator may need to understand a queuing study as used to evaluate options to resolve a patient waiting problem in emergency services?

ADDITIONAL RESOURCES

These references are recommended for additional reading and more comprehensive content beyond the scope of this book.

Barry, R., Murcko, A., Brubaker, C. (2002). The Six Sigma Book for Healthcare. Chicago: Health Administration Press.
Griffith, J., White, K. (2002). The Well-Managed Healthcare Organization. Chicago: Health Administration Press.
Harrell, C., Bateman, R., Gogg, T., Mott, J. (1996). System Improvement Using Simulation. Orem, UT: Promodel Corporation.
Longest, Jr., B., Rakich, J., Darr, K. (2004). Managing Health Services Organizations and Systems. Baltimore, MD: Health Professions Press.
Veney, J., Kaluzny, A. (1998). Evaluation and Decision Making for Health Services. Chicago: Health Administration Press.
Wan, T. (1995). Analysis and Evaluation of Health Care Systems: An Integrated Approach to Managerial Decision Making. Baltimore, MD: Health Professions Press.

CHAPTER 11

Process Simulation and Predictive Modeling

This chapter introduces process simulation and predictive modeling, especially these fundamental concepts:

- Essential tools and techniques
- Advancing from simple to sophisticated models
- Contemporary approaches to process modeling
- Using animation and integration in production applications

Simulation is a means of experimenting with a detailed model of real production processes or systems. The objective of these experiments or models is to determine how actual process or systems are likely to respond to change. These changes may involve modification to structure, components, sequencing, and other operations to understand and forecast expectations with some degree of certainty.

Process simulation and modeling of some type has been used in a variety of ways for many years. No one is absolutely sure when simple simulation and model-building techniques were developed. A fundamental principle as old as the scientific method itself is that symbolic representation leads to a clearer view of interactions among and within system components. In the context of healthcare delivery, simulation and modeling focus on operational components as combinations of process components (inputs, outputs, etc.) that interact to accomplish specific objectives.

Simulation enables analysts to study a defined set of components in a variety of combinations, permutations, durations, and sequences to understand and realistically forecast operational expectations with some degree of certainty.

These elements, in varying combinations, constitute a process or subsystem of yet a larger system. Components may be groups of professionals and administrative staff, instruments, equipment, information systems, other resources, facilities or policies. Each component controls some function or group of functions. Each function creates a product or service with some organizational value. Predictive modeling quantifies this value with expectations using simulation models with objectives defining forecast outcomes with varying degrees of certainty. By using increasingly powerful systems with virtually infinite capabilities, a model's precision and acceptable levels of forecast risk are easily modified. Iterative simulation runs generate years of expected operational activity in seconds. These results are used to study various options available to decision-makers.

Early simulation models were cumbersome and complex. Examples include nuclear chain reaction modeling during the Manhattan Project in the 1940s. Quantitative models were relatively small. Their limited size, complexity, computer resources, and research capabilities demanded larger data sets and calculation complexity. Because early limited computer capabilities affected a significant number of system parameters, requirements for more calculations rapidly became unmanageable. Although simulation uses in the Manhattan Project were well-known, they were not isolated examples. More recently, interest in simulation and process modeling has increased with these techniques recognized as vital tools to support digital healthcare process transformation. Most of this interest has been associated with increasing interest by healthcare organizations embracing QM, continuous process reengineering, Six Sigma, and Lean Enterprise initiatives.

For example, the physical facilities of a hospital, staff, physicians, administrative personnel, diagnostic instruments, and information systems are examples of relatively self-contained healthcare system components at one level and parts of a larger healthcare system at another level, possibly overall healthcare delivery in a city or county. All of these objects or organizations incorporate process (re)design and resource allocation decisions that can be supported by simulation and predictive modeling.

Dramatic increases in computer capabilities and other technological advances have made complex modeling feasible for practical applications. Navy medicine modeled Marine casualty intake and patient flow processes in a combat zone fleet hospital design during the 1980s by using large mainframe computers. Increasingly faster and more powerful desktop computer applications have made simulation capability more accessible and less costly. "Off-the-shelf" commercial simulation software is easier to use because it does not require expert-level competency in software programming or complex logic. Simulation capabilities became more robust as software and chip speed increased and more "on board memory" became commonplace. Modeling in support of strategic decision-making has incorporated animation of complex analyses, enabling decision-makers to better understand options or less expensive alternatives without detailed and technical burdens of complex analyses. Simulation and predictive modeling is increasingly popular and more recently the method of choice in process improvement, BPR, Six Sigma initiatives, and decision-support applications.

CREDIBILITY AND ACCEPTANCE

Managed care growth in the late 20th century focused on acceleration and escalation of healthcare costs. Model-building gained increasing acceptance to support more complex and increasingly more critical resource allocation decisions. Rigorous capital investment justification became necessary in order to acquire capital and respond to frequent human resource shortages.

Simulation and process modeling are now viewed by senior management as credible and reliable components of process improvement and more realistic forecasts of anticipated performance. Virtually all projects that merit serious study include model-building to better understand assumptions, underlying implications and expectations before approval. As in other industries, health care decision-making is no exception as more analytic and animated models demonstrate clinical, business, and management engineering principles. Additionally, computer hardware advances increased research capabilities to perform more calculations much faster with increasingly sophisticated capability. These powerful simulation characteristics advanced modeling capabilities to evaluate interaction variation and iteration performance. Ongoing enhancements resulted in more accurate models and substantial cost reduction to rapidly run and rerun models to simulate more options, resulting in better decision-making. These advances in computerized simulation capabilities led to more complex models using realistic activity representing systems, processes, and interactions rather than oversimplified abstractions.

As simulation engines of computers process vast amounts of data with speed and precision, dynamic modeling as a byproduct of actual production has enabled real-time assessment of all events. Computers keep each event in proper sequence and consider previously identified interdependencies far more effectively than any manual calculations conceived by research analysts. Models can evaluate even more complex and dynamic simulated systems in compressed time frames with continually enhanced capabilities. Learning curves for model-building and validation have been reduced from years and months to weeks, days, hours, minutes, and seconds. Simplifying assumptions and relative ease of use in Six Sigma initiatives encouraged senior management to consider simulated recommendations.

> Simulation is an ideal analytic tool when "pilot testing" is not practical to evaluate ideas and costly options. Simulation and model building are necessary when recommendations based solely on simple "average-based forecasting" are inadequate.

Model-building frames system components and variables in a quantified format that facilitates a better understanding of systems and process component interaction by teams and senior management. This increased comprehension and in-depth understanding of these complex interactions is enhanced in ways that were otherwise impractical. Simulation and modeling has improved forecasts credibly and reliability by predicting behaviors, especially in real-time production systems.

Simulation models:

- Predict outcomes of system modifications with action-based model prediction. Reliable prediction requires systematic learning about short-term and long-term alternative courses of action.
- Educate team members, senior management, and "process owners" about process modifications to identify alternative courses of action.
- Alternative actions are easily tested to determine effects as a prerequisite to implementation. Usually performing such tests on production systems are not feasible or too costly. Coupled with graphic animation, simulation illustrates both "current and proposed future state" workflow, process capability and capacity, productivity, and equipment utilization throughout a system.
- Are advanced, robust, and powerful problem-solving tools and techniques.
- Enable analysts to answer important questions.
- Define an idea with quantified expected impacts.
- Use animation options to "sell a solution" to skeptical decision-makers by fostering optimism and a "let's try it and see" attitude.

That said, simpler tools and techniques provide adequate answers faster and at lower cost in some situations. Even when computers and other resources are available to analyze every possible detail in every process in a system, time and cost required to build and validate a simulation model may not justify expected analytical outcomes.

Most healthcare systems are both dynamic and stochastic. A dynamic system implies predictable action in response to varying influences that change over time. For example, changes in patient arrival rates, equipment, facility availability and staffing levels vary dynamically or stochastically. Stochastic variability suggests indiscriminate or random change. Models of various types are used to identify, validate, and test potential process or system improvements and to remediate problems in either dynamic or stochastic systems.

MODEL TYPES

Simulation of healthcare delivery process or system changes can use these common models:

- *Opinion models* using single equations and variables are constants that are developed from activity averages. These models are composed primarily of individual or group assumptions, beliefs, and ideas of system representatives. Occasionally, these models degenerate into a test of egos rather than solutions because little if any quantifiable data are used to evaluate alternatives.
- *Static mathematical models* arithmetically emulate a system with operational characteristics described with equations that define implications of options or alternatives. Spreadsheet analyses are examples of static mathematical models that determine expected system behavior and performance by summing individual effects. More complex spreadsheet models use macros and other spreadsheet functions that incorporate repetitive capabilities.
- *Simulation models* are event-driven mathematical and probability-based using equations to express existing or proposed operational characteristics. An event is anything that happens at a certain point in time (an emergency room patient arriving for urgent unscheduled emergent care).

Event occurrence changes variables in potentially complex arithmetic and statistical computations. Risk analysis and probability-driven computations forecast occurrences, responses, and observations of occurrences for a potentially large number of events iteratively over time to emulate variable system behaviors and performance. Multiple iterations of expectations can be rapidly analyzed with time compression capabilities to develop a range of expected outcomes rather than mean-based point estimates. Even inexpensive commercial simulation tools include animation capabilities to graphically depict alternative scenarios.

Actual systems or process activities do not exhibit identical behaviors with every occurrence. Therefore models that are based on average activity cannot reliably emulate or forecast these activities.

Control modules in leading healthcare information systems can process real-time outcomes or impacts of events such as instrument downtime, transport failures, and unforeseen or other less-than-ideal situations with some degree of certainty. The potential for variation increases dramatically (usually exponentially), when human behavior and associated factors are included. These very dynamic variations are most difficult to replicate. Simulation models are unique decision-support tools with the capability to emulate these variations. Reliable predictive models simulate the complicated behaviors and generate credible forecasts that demonstrate process influence, impacts, and system performance.

Gaining insight to cause-and-effect relationships and their magnitude is difficult because simulation complexity increases exponentially with each additional system variable and escalates even faster with interdependencies. These problems are common in both dynamic and stochastic models. They also complicate decision-maker analysis of simulations as the number of variables and interrelationships multiply. Figure 11.1 illustrates this complexity correlation by depicting the abstraction of the degree of difficulty of model design and output analysis. A model's underlying structure grows incrementally more difficult as each additional variable is added.

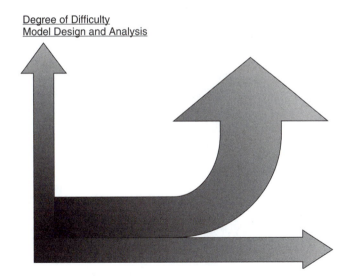

FIGURE 11.1   Analytical difficulty versus number of variables.

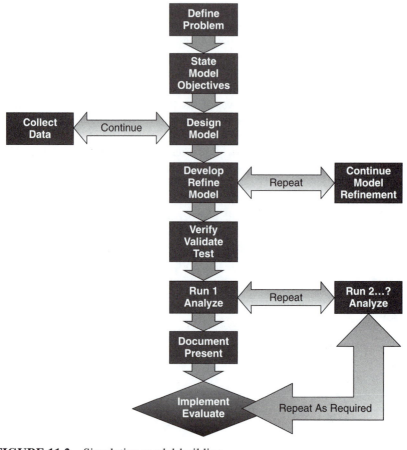

FIGURE 11.2   Simulation model-building.

DEGREE OF DIFFICULTY: MODEL DESIGN AND ANALYSIS

Insight and benefit gained from models correlate closely to the emulation capability of the model. This emulation capability is measured by the extent to which a model produces expected responses for a process or system. Simulation models produce more dynamic and stochastic emulations of process or system behaviors. Simulation models more realistically reflect actual system or process capability compared with static mathematic or opinion-based models. Simulation accounts for the effects of variance that actually occur in a process or system. In this context, variance implies that change occurs from one incident to another. Traditional static mathematic models and analytical methods do not effectively address this variation because their performance calculations are derived from constants based on averages. *Performance computations based solely on a mean do not account for variance.* Erroneous conclusions are likely if this limitation is not recognized.

Model definition and design have evolved and are more intuitive as model-building terminology and logic become more familiar to "systems savvy" management engineers, systems and operations analysts. As these simulators became available and user-friendly, they became popular in progressive healthcare organizations. Simulators are common in undergraduate classes, especially in courses or projects where simulation is one of many research techniques taught or utilized. Widespread adoption of graphic user interfaces and web browsers has evolved and is now commonplace in healthcare-specific applications, including department-specific templates. This tool, as with other third- and fourth-generation products, incorporates user-friendly animation capabilities as well as automatically generated statistical reporting of key statistics for each iterative simulation run. Figure 11.2 is a flowchart summarizing simulation and predictive model-building techniques discussed in this chapter.

SUMMARY

This chapter introduced and discussed simulation and predictive modeling terminology, tools, techniques, and concepts.

Fundamental concepts and content focused on

- Advancing from simple to sophisticated models
- Contemporary approaches to process modeling
- Using animation and integration in production applications

CHAPTER QUESTIONS

These questions reinforce student understanding, learning, and retention while stimulating class discussion:

1. Explain the differences between static, dynamic, and simulation models.
2. Describe the most important reason to use simulation rather than mean-based approaches to predictive modeling.
3. How does animation improve simulation capabilities?
4. Why is including variable variation in predictive models important?
5. How does changing the number of variables or the relationship between variables affect modeling?

ADDITIONAL RESOURCES

These references are recommended for additional reading and more comprehensive content beyond the scope of this book.

Barry, R., Murcko, A., Brubaker, C. (2002). The Six Sigma Book for Healthcare. Chicago: Health Administration Press.

Griffith, J., White, K. (2002). The Well-Managed Healthcare Organization. Chicago: Health Administration Press.

Harrell, C., Bateman, R., Gogg, T., Mott, J. (1996). System Improvement Using Simulation. Orem, UT: Promodel Corporation.

Larson, J. (2001). Management Engineering. Chicago: Healthcare Information and Management Systems Society.

Longest, Jr., B., Rakich, J., Darr, K. (2004). Managing Health Services Organizations and Systems. Baltimore, MD: Health Professions Press.

CHAPTER 12

Strategic Application of Six Sigma Concepts

This chapter introduces Six Sigma fundamentals and relationships to QM and BPR principles by focusing on these key concepts:

- Multifaceted and multidimensional definitions
- DMAIC strategies
- Benchmarking and breakthrough fundamentals
- Six Sigma business case

Six Sigma concepts embrace multifaceted aspects and multidimensional components. These fundamental components are appropriate in any organization, at any time, for any purpose, and with any audience. Six Sigma had its origins within General Electric (GE). Healthcare providers only adopted these concepts within the last decade.

DMAIC

- **D**efining, articulating, and deploying plans to realize sustainable improvement.
- **M**easuring systems and applications achieve plans by knowing what to measure, how to measure properly, and obtain commitment to pursue corrective measurements and support appropriate remedial action derived from analysis associated with these measures.

- Analyzing system, application, or process performance gaps against benchmarks and then diagnosing capability measures and assessing performance gaps to uncover "solutions" that more successful organizations use to operate at higher Six Sigma levels.
- Improving system, application, and process elements to achieve performance goals by defining and using metrics to analyze data and then defining and prioritizing remediation actions.
- Controlling system-level critical characteristics that add value and then monitoring changes and incorporating "audits" to sustain these critical value-adding performance characteristics.

Just as Edward Deming is acknowledged as the "father" of QM and statistical process control in Japanese manufacturing settings, so is Jack Welsh the acknowledged father of Six Sigma while he led General Electric Corporation (GE). Since then, Six Sigma has evolved, has been enhanced, and is widely adopted in manufacturing. More recently, these principles were modified and refined for service settings, including health care.

Regardless of which perspective is the focus of any organizational transformation, Six Sigma thinking requires the organization's leadership to rethink strategy from tracking average performance to benchmarking against each patient's optimal expectation. For example, rather than track a patient's average length of stay in an emergency department, Six Sigma organizations track the percentage of emergency stays less than 150 minutes, striving to drive this metric to a Six Sigma level.

Table 12.1 characterizes these metrics for healthcare provider goal-setting. Community hospitals typically operate at Six Sigma level 2, whereas more progressive pioneering organizations that are initially investing in Six Sigma initiatives are likely to be at Six Sigma level 3.

As an organization monitors key metrics, a number of other patient-centric impacts are evaluated as a consequence of striving to achieve improved Six Sigma performance.

For example, patient waiting times before and during each emergent visit are reduced, potentially lowering departmental staffing requirements as "perceived workload" drops. Reduced "cycle times" generate cost savings by decreasing direct labor time requirements. Some providers have reduced waiting area sizes and used this space for other more productive programs. Because of high construction and maintenance costs, any process improvement that yields space savings or cost avoidance of new construction is very desirable.

Early in Six Sigma initiatives, quality professionals, systems analysts, management engineers, operations analysts, software engineers, and IT professionals are

TABLE 12.1   Six Sigma by the Numbers

Sigma Level	Quality Yield	Cost of Quality
2	69.0%	Uncompetitive
3	93.3%	25–40%
4	99.4%	15–25%
5	99.8%	5–15%
6	99.99997%	World class

expected to demonstrate core competencies to be "credentialed" as Green, Black, and even Master Black Belt experts. These digital transformationalists demonstrate increased process improvement competencies as they move up Six Sigma levels:

- Technical and analytic capabilities
- Project management experience
- Team facilitation and leadership

Figure 12.1 depicts a common Six Sigma initiatives' organizational structure and deployment of key participants.

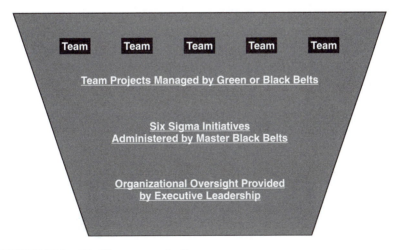

FIGURE 12.1   Six Sigma organization.

Figure 12.2 highlights these levels within a provider organization when Six Sigma principles are applied in an enterprise-wide deployment. Allocation of recourses at the business or process level is required so that adequate analytic and implementation expertise is applied to each operation or task.

Six Sigma deployment strategies and breakthrough expectations are formulated and communicated by senior leaders to understand key differences between traditional process improvement thinking, techniques, and tools as initial Six Sigma thinking. These strategies are developed and executed at the leadership level and deployed throughout all divisions and departments of an IDS.

These organizational and structural changes and actions are necessary to build from a solid foundation that supports rigorous analysis and iterative experimentation to advance to and function at higher levels of Six Sigma performance.

Six Sigma is recognized as an important tool to drive out medical errors and reduce unnecessary delays while recovering costs lost to poor quality. Because, as an industry, health care is a late adopter, providers are benefiting from experiences in other service industries that required substantial conceptual changes in traditional Six Sigma methodologies. Key components of these Six Sigma deployment and breakthrough strategies are as follows:

- Recognize
- Define
- Measure

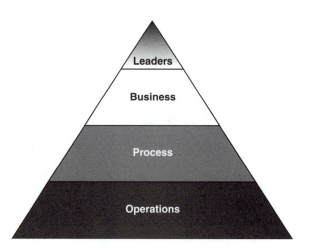

FIGURE 12.2   Strategic levels of Six Sigma organization and impact.

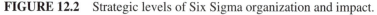

- Analyze
- Improve
- Control
- Standardize
- Integrate

Leaders must understand that effective deployment of these methodologies requires a strategic commitment to organizational realignment, adequate infrastructure development, system mapping, key driver determination, and results tracking. These sometimes subtle and other times more radical modifications are necessary to ensure that Six Sigma initiatives are tailored to operate effectively within each organization's unique culture.

For example, leaders need to develop, articulate, and reinforce a 3-year core process strategy that involves goals for quality and cost recovery. This comprehensive approach embodies simultaneous deployment of several process transformations within an orderly strategic framework. This disciplined approach prevents a "project-by-project" mindset common among IT professionals.

To avoid unnecessary complications, these lessons learned from other healthcare transformation pioneers should be used:

- *Identify* early clinical improvement opportunities
- *Analyze* DRG data in collaboration with benchmarking partners
- *Focus* on areas like those with proven Six Sigma successes in pioneering organizations

Many organizations purchase comparative data from commercial sources (Solucient, Premier, Applied Management Services, Caldwell & Associates, Barrick & Associates, and Data Advantage). These consulting groups, data vendors, and information brokers specialize in identifying peer organizations, goal-setting, and process redesign and in leading effective Six Sigma and related transformation initiatives.

Specialized expertise will be required and should be carefully targeted, using internal and external expertise.

- Project management and disciplined action planning
- Matching staffing to demand and shaping demand
- Medication safety
- Advancing accelerated cost reduction
- Strategic guidance and critical considerations

As Six Sigma concepts are applied, they require definition in ways that prepare project teams and senior leaders to understand and apply tools and techniques appropriately. This approach to breakthrough performance improvement embraces a quality focus. This focus adds clarity to unnecessary process variation, develops and implements countermeasures and solutions to avoid unproductive variation.

While achieving breakthrough quality improvement is the primary goal, eliminating waste and reducing cost are secondary beneficial byproducts. Team leaders and members should understand that an expected "breakthrough" improvement is necessary because an existing process is so broken that less intensive, less rigorous, and incremental improvements quality management (QM), Business process reengineering (BPR) or continuous process improvement (CPI) are inadequate.

Breakthrough improvement requires significant investments in labor and innovative, disruptive technology. In addition to rigorous qualitative and quantitative analysis, organizational belief systems must be transformed with organizational energies instilling a momentum for change and intense focus on significantly transforming each mission critical process. Without belief system transformation, sustainable performance improvement is unlikely. Tactically, a quantitative definition expresses Six Sigma solutions as a "world class" achievement. In the Six Sigma context, "world class" means a sustainable process transformation resulting in less than 3.4 errors or defects per million opportunities. Current healthcare processes operate at Six Sigma levels 2 and 3.

From yet another perspective, Six Sigma strategically focuses rigorous analytics and performance benchmarks with measures for each mission critical process. This assessment compares current capability and process performance with a statistically valid ideal process. After process transformation is implemented, monitoring continues to sustain achievements that perpetuate, reduce process variation and eliminate waste.

Table 12.2 introduces DMAIC as a mnemonic with analytic parallels between key aspects of Six Sigma methodology to those discussed earlier as strategies and tactical approaches to QM deployment and process reengineering.

This mnemonic is quite similar in content and context as espoused by Deming, Labowitz, and others which were explained in chapter 6.

- **D**efine what plans must be in place to realize sustainable improvement
- **M**easure business systems supporting plans
- **A**nalyze gaps in system performance against comparable credible benchmarks
- **I**mprove system elements to achieve performance goals
- **C**ontrol system-level value-critical characteristics

Table 12.2 also compares DMAIC, Focus-PCDA, and FADE.

TABLE 12.2   Six Sigma and QM Mnemonics

Six Sigma	Deming: Focus-PCDA	QM Labowitz: FADE
Define	**P**lan	**F**ocus
Measure	**C**ontrol	**A**nalyze
Analyze	**D**evelop	**D**evelop
Improve	**A**ssess	**E**xecute
Control		

DMAIC

- **D**efining, articulating, and deploying plans to realize sustainable improvement.
- **M**easuring systems and applications achieve plans by knowing what to measure, how to measure properly, and obtain commitment to pursue corrective measurements and support appropriate remedial action derived from analysis associated with these measures.
- **A**nalyzing system, application, or process performance gaps against benchmarks and then diagnosing capability measures and assessing performance gaps to uncover "solutions" that more successful organizations use to operate at higher Six Sigma levels.
- **I**mproving system, application, and process elements to achieve performance goals by defining and using metrics to analyze data and then defining and prioritizing remediation actions.
- **C**ontrolling system-level critical characteristics that add value and then monitoring changes and incorporating "audits" to sustain these critical value-adding performance characteristics.

Table 12.3 succinctly explains these concepts with terminology focusing on the process level in any healthcare provider organization. Six Sigma DMAIC principles can be applied at a provider's organization, operations, business and process level.

DMAIC tools and techniques are focused on problematic dysfunctional processes. These processes have eroded quality and/or unacceptably high cost. Frequently, these problems are linked to other operational issues. When broken down, processes

TABLE 12.3   Process Level Application of DMAIC

- *Define* process contributing to problems to determine if problems are functionally related to personnel, products, service, transaction, or environment.

- *Create* process maps that break down key processes into unique steps, events, or activities, and then effectively search for solutions to each identified problem.

- *Measure* capability of each process, determining operational leverage of each process while identifying and separating value-added from non–value-added activities.

- *Analyze* data to identify relevant trends and prevalent patterns between and among process variables to identify improvement drivers.

- *Improve* product and service characteristics for each process by screening variables and ranking those of most impact to establish operating specifications.

- *Control* process variables by reducing those exerting unnecessary, undue, inappropriate, or unwarranted influence.

---

include errors that reflect interrelated problems and causes. Because of the hierarchical nature of these process problems, Six Sigma initiatives target system interfaces and handoffs from one task to another at the process level.

Operational problems often reflect dissonance from broken links between patient satisfaction and organizational profitability. DMAIC applications at this level define contributing problems to determine how these problems are related to personnel, products, services, or transactions. By creating process maps, analysts break down these processes into individual steps, events, or activities and then identify potential solutions.

DMAIC metrics identify opportunities to understand, integrate then leverage process performance. Analyses focus on information and data to assess patterns and trends in order to determine relationships between and among each process variable. DMAIC objectives at this level include process transformation to measurably improve patient services in these key processes. By screening for variables offering significant potential, solutions are developed to reestablish higher operating specifications at a higher Six Sigma level. These solutions must demonstrate sustainable consistency with less process variation (increased control of variables), exerting a positive impact on desirable patient-centric needs and expectations.

Operations level breakthrough strategies develop as transformation exposes "operational issues" as collections of higher level problems confounded by some organizational dysfunction.

Six Sigma strategies require analysis to break down each "systems and processes issue" into component parts. This breakdown allows problems to be defined and action plans to be devised, ultimately producing positive action. Usually, operational dysfunction is attributed to ineffectively linked systems, applications, processes, or tasks.

Tactical solutions usually resolve problematic support systems. For example, a quality information system reports only statistical data on defects that can only be resolved retrospectively. Recognizing that these findings are likely, managers must carefully focus on mission critical operations level Six Sigma initiatives. Project teams must be tasked to identify, establish, test, and refine Six Sigma performance standards to measure different dimensions of each expected improvement. Ongoing tracking reduces variance and consistently demonstrates improved, sustained process performance. Teams must continue to refine and "fine-tune" standards to maintain acceptance by key stakeholders and to sustain "process owner" credibility to be relevant, equitable, and achievable. Then and only then should focus shift to seamless integration of these performance standards and expectations into policies and procedures.

This process of institutionalizing improved performance and practice into day-to-day operations is accomplished by interweaving transformed processes and practices into standard operating policies and procedures. Digitally transformed care delivery systems, applications, processes, and related operational tasks visibly demonstrate consistently improved performance. Six Sigma sponsors must continually reinforce and reward breakthrough performance with tangible rewards and recognition. Process owners and key stakeholders must stay motivated to reach even higher levels of achievement.

For example, GE ties 40% of each manager's annual incentive compensation to their capability to achieve and sustain measurable progress toward world class Six Sigma quality. Six Sigma leaders throughout each GE operating unit, including managers and vice presidents, recognize that motivation is highest when success is acknowledged while understanding that there is an inherent permission to fail. Improvements are more likely to be incorporated into critical business strategies when key managers' compensation and annual performance evaluations are tied to successful implementation and sustained performance as incentives. Breakthrough strategies are achieved when Six Sigma strategies are identified, applied, and implemented as unique phases with key milestones over mutually agreed upon timelines. Senior management should use relevant and proven tactics to keep each Six Sigma initiative focused on achievement of realistic expectations throughout each phase of digital process transformation. Strategically timed milestones are necessary to track each initiative's progress.

Six Sigma leaders must view mistakes as tools for personal and organization growth.

Leaders must ensure that relevant benchmarks are embedded into transformed processes by continuous comparison with pioneering competitors (compare organizational processes with best practice). Consistently using comparative benchmarking data facilitates realistic goal-setting to achieve improved quality, cost reduction, and faster cycle times.

As a Six Sigma initiative matures from initial chartering to implemented recommendations, sponsors must monitor project status quantitatively in both absolute and relative terms. Oversight must periodically require data analysis at appropriate levels. Ideally, data collection and analyses should be a natural byproduct of milestone achievement to avoid otherwise redundant reporting requirements, which may slow this progress. Periodic oversight by senior executive sponsors should focus on high-level tracking of performance to established objectives and action plans to target dates. Gantt charts are best used for this purpose and should be prepared to facilitate periodic progress reporting by project sponsors. Tracking reports should incorporate relevant metrics that highlight planned actual task completion, cost, timing, and net savings as well as interim achievement, especially when related to quality improvement. This reporting should incorporate classic project management principles without micromanagement as discussed in Chapter 7.

As Six Sigma initiatives are in progress, analysts should be striving to identify and then standardize systems to specifications that have proven to be "best in class." This benchmarking compares performance with benchmarked processes in those organizations recognized for "best practice" capabilities by routinely demonstrating sustained optimal performance.

Benchmarking

Focus on world class performance to continuously compare mission critical processes both internally and with pioneering competitors' best practice by measuring customer loyalty, service, market share, and cost.

As these performance improvements are implemented in all venues throughout the IDS, leaders must challenge teams involved in digital process transformation to emulate and integrate these "best-in-class" processes and systems into an IDS-wide strategic planning infrastructure. Strategies and tactics should be built into future design and then monitored for timely achievement of action-oriented objectives. By expecting that desired results are routinely being integrated into day-to-day process and practices, these objectives will be achieved as envisioned and sustainable realization. Recognizing that each tactic is composed of key characteristics, each should be incorporated in an actionable checklist to guide a project team through this disciplined Six Sigma process.

Table 12.4 is an example of a checklist that can be adapted to include unique organizational cultural characteristics and specific terminology understandable by all team members.

Strategic breakthroughs actually occur at three levels in a healthcare provider organization. Business is the highest level, which encompasses all activities related to organization-wide impacts. Operations is the next level, and process is the lowest

TABLE 12.4   Successful Six Sigma Deployment Checklist

Identify, recognize, and define:

Understand fundamental concepts and recognize breakthrough strategy as a problem-solving methodology with unique tools.

Recognize profitability impact of process by defining mission critical processes.

Appreciate that a key component is variation across processes that impact results, e.g., cost, cycle time, and defect rates.

Characterize, measure, and analyze:

Consider process status as measured and identify goals by establishing baselines and benchmarks.

Provide a starting point to measure improvement.

Create an action plan to close gap between "current state" and desired "future state" processes.

Break down every process into key characteristics with fundamentally unique components.

Create a detailed description of each step in a process.

Measure process capabilities to optimize, improve, and control:

Identify steps required to improve each process and reduce major variation sources.

Identify key process variables through statistically designed experiments, and then target and isolate "vital few" with greatest impact using Pareto principles.

Use knowledge gained to improve and control processes, thereby improving patient satisfaction and stakeholder value as well as organization's profitability.

Standardize, integrate, and institutionalize:

Emphasize Six Sigma integration, not just QM, BPR, and CPI project focus.

Articulate impact on collective high-level mission critical performance as outcomes of smaller projects.

level of Six Sigma initiatives' planning, deployment, and expected impact. Business, operations, and process level impacts are unique and occur in different ways.

When chartering a Six Sigma initiative, senior leaders and mid-level managers must be aware of and sensitive to strategic requirements for effective change management. An organization's leader is accountable for business level impacts. Senior management team members administer operations level impacts, whereas department directors manage process level achievements. Six Sigma impacts at a business or organizational level are focused on strategic results that can reasonably be expected to make significant improvements in an organization's digital transformation, informational, and economic systems (e.g., patient care, internal and external customer feedback, or supplier quality) (Figure 12.3).

Leaders must understand that several years of a high level of commitment are required to consistently recognize and experience a Six Sigma success. Consistent and committed oversight is required to achieve a successful transformation of this magnitude. Although constant commitment is essential, significant improvement in quality and profitability, as with other critical mission driven processes, is incrementally achieved. Throughout this extended period of time, consistent application of Six Sigma principles and rigorous analytic methodologies must be dynamic and fluid to experience change demonstrated by quantifiably improved effectiveness at all organizational levels. Because extended periods of transformation are expected, senior leaders should be cautious about beginning an initiative of this magnitude if a change in executive management is anticipated.

The business case for the significant investment of time and organizational resources in Six Sigma is appropriate. This case is founded on Edward Deming's rationale that statistical process control is the basis for all performance improvement to be realized from digital transformation of healthcare delivery processes. As sustained control over process variation is improved and consistently demonstrated, significant error reduction occurs. With this error reduction improved quality of care delivery is achieved and cost savings result. Figure 12.4 graphically

Future State Six Sigma Level
World Class Health Care
Decreased Process Variation Yields Increase Performance At Less Cost

FIGURE 12.3   Perspective of process variation after Six Sigma application: World class health care.

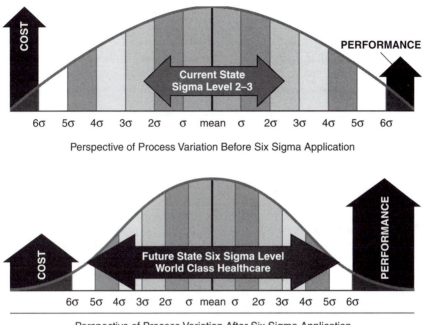

Perspective of Process Variation Before Six Sigma Application

Perspective of Process Variation After Six Sigma Application
World Class Healthcare

FIGURE 12.4 Six Sigma business case: Classic bell curve as discussed in control charts construction concepts.

depicts this rationale as a business case for Six Sigma application to digitally transform mission critical processes in a patient-centric care delivery system. With effective IT application, process transformation and critical performance variability are substantially reduced with more control. With reduced variation, increased process capability and consistency are experienced. As depicted, as distance from a process performance mean to Six Sigma (6σ) is reduced, higher quality at lower cost is achieved.

When healthcare delivery process performance increases from Six Sigma Level 2+ with 25% error rates and 30% excess cost to Six Sigma Level 6 (i.e., approximately one error per million occurrences with virtually no excess cost), patients experience world class health care. This is the goal of digital transformation with Six Sigma "by the numbers."

SUMMARY

This chapter introduced and discussed important terminology, tools, techniques, and concepts detailing how Six Sigma principles are applicable in healthcare provider organizations.

Fundamental concepts and content focused on

- Multifaceted and multidimensional definitions
- DMAIC strategies
- Benchmarking and breakthrough fundamentals
- Business case for Six Sigma

CHAPTER QUESTIONS

These questions reinforce student understanding, learning, and retention while stimulating class discussion:

1. Succinctly state the business base for Six Sigma in healthcare provider organizations.
2. Identify what the mnemonics Focus-PCDA, FADE, and DMAIC mean and explain how these approaches are similar and different.
3. What is meant by Six Sigma strategic business, process, and operations levels? Describe how DMAIC is applied at each level.
4. How is a classic bell curve related to standardized deviations used to determine UCL and LCL in control charts?
5. How is QM related to Six Sigma principles?
6. How are GE, Toyota, and Japanese manufacturing organizations related to Deming, Ishikawa, and Jack Welch?
7. Identify four core elements of a successful Six Sigma deployment plan and explain several key components of each phase.
8. Describe what is meant by multifaceted and multidimensional and identify key aspects of each dimension.
9. How are QM, BPR, and Six Sigma similar and how are they different?

ADDITIONAL RESOURCES

These references are recommended for additional reading and more comprehensive content beyond the scope of this book.

Barry, R., Murcko, A., Brubaker, C. (2002). The Six Sigma Book for Healthcare. Chicago: Health Administration Press.

Larson, J. (2001). Management Engineering. Chicago: Healthcare Information and Management Systems Society.

CHAPTER 13

Lean Enterprise Theory and Facilitation

This chapter introduces Lean enterprise theory with facilitation tools and techniques, building on relationships to QM, BPR, and Six Sigma principles discussed in other chapters.

Lean enterprise theory embraces these key concepts:

- Lean enterprise metrics
- Strategies, tools, and principles that increase efficiency, decrease waste, and improve quality
- Value stream mapping (VSM) and visual management
- Error-proofing and standardizing operations
- Push versus pull systems and "takt" time

Lean enterprise strategies are being emulated in health care after demonstrating positive outcomes in other service industries. Lean principles, specifically in automotive companies like Toyota, were recognized as being useful in improving virtually any process or system (automobile production or patient healthcare delivery). As Lean principles are embraced and applied throughout any organization, significant cost reduction, waste elimination, increased patient satisfaction, and personnel effectiveness are achieved.

This concept of "lean management" or "Lean thinking" is most commonly associated with Japanese thinking based on inspiration from quality guru W. Edwards Deming. Lean thinking means using less to do more, faster.

Deming and other QM devotees taught organizational leaders and operations managers to stop depending on cumbersome and often redundant inspections to achieve quality. Instead, by focusing on continuous process improvement, quality is built into consistant service with minimal variation. Lean thinking has not been embraced in health care as in organizations where waste of time, money, supplies, and goodwill is openly acknowledged. Lean management works in health care in much the same way as in other industries based on early adopter experience.

A strong consensus is building among healthcare leaders that Lean principles are effective in reducing pervasive waste throughout America's healthcare delivery and financing systems, processes, and practice. The Institute for Healthcare Improvement (IHI) is championing adoption of Lean management strategies while challenging healthcare providers to improve processes and outcomes, reduce cost, and increase patient, provider, and employee satisfaction. Figure 13.1 depicts expected outcomes of effective lean deployment.

Lean goals focus on digital transformation of outdated legacy systems, usually requiring replacement with state-of-art "Lean systems." Effective systematic digital transformation improves process efficiency, organizational performance, and effectiveness by eliminating waste, reducing delays, and costs, and improving quality. The consistency of patient-centric healthcare delivery and the competency of organizations and individual providers are improved by conforming to standards that meet or exceed patients' needs and expectations.

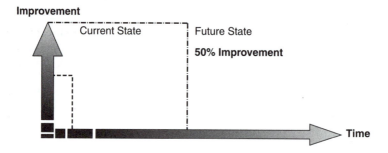

FIGURE 13.1   Lean process improvement expectations over time.

Lean achievements experienced at Virginia Mason Medical Center in Seattle, an early adopter, include:

- Demonstratively better patient satisfaction
- Avoidance of $6 million in budgeted capital investments
- Reallocation of 13,000 square feet of expensive space upon process redesign
- Reduction in inventory costs by more than $350,000 per year
- Decrease in infection rates
- Reduced staff travel time

VISUAL MANAGEMENT

Lean concepts stress VSM and visual management to highlight and focus relevant resources on opportunities by visualizing process or system elements from input to output through key aspects of value transformation. VSM is similar in concept, use, and creation to flowcharting and documenting workflow for work simplification, to change an existing process. All team members must understand a process or system from beginning to end, not only those aspects of the process that affect them, for a team to produce credible recommendations.

Figure 13.2 is an example of a VSM used to expedite and improve emergency workflow by resequencing ordering of authorized standard orders to an earlier point in the process. This change has been successfully adopted by emergency physicians and nursing staff for common high-volume procedures when an experienced triage nurse can correctly anticipate and initiate accepted physician diagnostics. This change dramatically shortens patient wait time and staff under-utilization until diagnostic procedures have been completed and reported to the physician for patient treatment.

Another example of a VSM of supply process flow begins when a product is received from a supplier through delivery and administration to patients. Transformation of product and service inputs into outputs is achieved by incorporating transformational information flow from input through output. An even more comprehensive VSM incorporates charging each supply item to a patient's account and replenishing item inventory by generating a purchase order to supply delivery from a preferred vendor.

VSM shows personnel, material, and information flows required to deliver patient care while distinguishing between value-added and non–value-added steps. This strategy and these methods have been successfully adapted to patient care in a variety of venues. Application of Lean techniques is enabling hospitals and clinics to streamline operations by focusing scarce and expensive resources on value as perceived by patients.

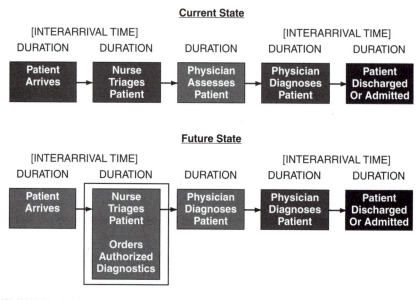

FIGURE 13.2   Emergency department VSM example.

Opportunities to deploy lean strategies in healthcare provider organizations are virtually everywhere:

- *Addressing* medication delivery and administration delays for pharmacy patients
- *Decreasing* caregiver travel time and distance
- *Eliminating*, *reducing*, or *automating* paperwork

As lean concepts are introduced, an organization should first focus on mission critical processes with lots of opportunities. Lean implementation is especially effective in conjunction with Six Sigma, BPR, or QM initiatives already targeted or underway. This strategy paces analysts and reinforces focus on value-added activities and material flow through care delivery processes to patients.

"Pull" rather than "push" transformation system design is encouraged to improve care delivery pace and associated processes.

Value streaming is used to optimize "takt" time (available work time) and to better match care delivery to patient demand requirements.

PULL, PUSH, AND TAKT TIME

Lean strategy incorporates a unique concept of "pull versus push" systems and processes. This approach has advantages that should be considered as new systems and processes are designed, developed, and implemented or as legacy systems are improved or redesigned.

Pull systems are more efficient and effective because non–value-added steps, such as waiting and transporting "handoffs," are excluded or eliminated. Common examples of these inefficiencies include

- System or personnel downtime
- Unproductive movement or travel of unnecessary distance between steps
- Unnecessary inspection or rework

Pull systems promptly deliver more care, service, and products more promptly and only when and as requested by "downstream" processes or requirements. Pull systems reflect a streamlined flow of patient care services with more efficient delivery than push processes.

Alternatively, push systems incorporate more inefficient components characterized by risky but required care delivery processes that hand off activities to downstream processes. Each handoff has a high potential for error or delay. These handoffs may result in unnecessary inventory or workload imbalance that generates costly idle resources or overtime.

Improvement teams must determine potential opportunities (acceptable "takt" times), in care delivery processes and related system components to achieve expected performance goals. Takt time represents a rate at which healthcare provider systems and processes must operate to meet demand requirements. When takt times are unacceptable because of time and distance observations, quantum advances in care delivery processes, diagnostic procedures, and therapies are unlikely to be achievable.

Visual management tools expose waste and encourage elimination and prevention from recurrence. Clear, concise communication and reinforcement of operational standards improves worksite efficiency throughout an IDS.

LEAN IMPLEMENTATIONS AND IMPLICATIONS

Effective implementation of visual management tools and techniques require:

- *Organizing* by using the "5 S's":
  - Sorting
  - Shining
  - Setting in order
  - Standardizing
  - Sustaining

- *Ensuring* effective task execution by displaying work standards at each work site
- Controlling processes by exposing and stopping errors
- Applying relevant counter-measures to prevent recurrence of resolved errors

Service and product quality is sustained when staff members strive to prevent or detect errors before they occur and are empowered to respond to errors with real-time resolution. Developing and sustaining this organizational philosophy requires consistent, deliberate, and visible leadership coupled with unwavering insistence that middle management "walks the talk" and maintains standards for zero tolerance of errors, defects, or waste.

Lean strategy incorporates embedded error-proofing technique as a structured approach in workflow design. This approach ensures quality care delivery throughout entire processes by encouraging providers to discover error sources in each component of workflow by using problem-solving techniques (cause and effect diagramming).

This technique does not focus on identifying and counting defects, but rather striving to eliminate error causes. In this context, an error is any deviation from specified delivery standards or clinical pathways. Errors cause defects and represent care delivery, products, or services that do not conform to patient expectations or requirements. Recognizing that defects are errors, error-proofing objectives focus on creating and sustaining an error-free care delivery culture in which defects are eliminated when identified and removing root causes of error.

Lean thinking considers waste as any unnecessary patient waiting, transport, and overproduction that should be radically reduced or eliminated. Labowitz, Caldwell and others refer to such unnecessary excess as "gold-plating" a process as discussed in Chapter 5.

In this context, waste includes any elements in process delivery of quality products and services that do not add measurable value. As excess activity is eliminated, inventory is reduced and inherently error-prone motions are minimized. Process lead and cycle times from task start to finish are optimized by reducing batch processing delays. Variable and fixed costs are reduced through targeted pricing and costing as well as value engineering and activity-based costing.

Waste, redundancies, errors, and escalating costs are pervasive in health care. Proven Lean tools and principles increase efficiency, decrease waste of costly scarce resources, and improve quality, as demonstrated in other service industries. Specifically, Lean implementations in health care enable providers to lower cost and improve quality of patient care delivery. As with other concepts discussed in this textbook, Lean enterprise tools and techniques often reflect little more than an organized and disciplined application of common sense.

Common sources of waste or error targeted by Lean strategies include human errors, methods, measurements, supplies, equipment, instruments, information technologies, and work environment. Table 13.1 highlights classic examples of these error sources; identifying error sources is a required prerequisite to developing and sustaining use of counter-measures as an effective outcome of classic Lean enterprise initiatives. Resolution requires acknowledgment that 85% of care process errors are most often caused by improper task, technology, or process design and less often by faulty worker execution or decision-making.

Early adopter organizations enjoy effective digital transformation of patient care delivery with quantum advances in diagnostic and therapeutic care. A compelling case to replace legacy systems is made when Lean principles are applied with patient-centric vision. Historically, multi-disciplinary initiatives that were staffed with information systems designers, operations analysts, and management engineers were not chartered to produce integrated "future state" solutions. These projects did little to eliminate delivery system shortcomings or to add real value from IT investments.

TABLE 13.1   Error Sources in Healthcare Delivery

Human errors

- Sensory overload
- Mental errors
- Mechanical process errors
- Distractions
- Memory loss
- Emotional control loss

Process errors

- Steps or sequence
- Patients or personnel movement, including transport
- Material, IT, information, technology, or patient movement
- Patient care or delivery process decision-making:
  - Who
  - What
  - Where
  - When
  - How
- Error-prone inspections

LEAN OPPORTUNITIES AND PRINCIPLED APPLICATION

Resources are best used by using Lean techniques to target problematic legacy systems. In Lean language, "Red flag" conditions are those with a high probability of error. These common "systemic" problems are usually obvious to an objective observer.

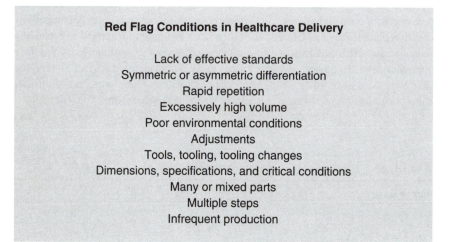

Red Flag Conditions in Healthcare Delivery

Lack of effective standards
Symmetric or asymmetric differentiation
Rapid repetition
Excessively high volume
Poor environmental conditions
Adjustments
Tools, tooling, tooling changes
Dimensions, specifications, and critical conditions
Many or mixed parts
Multiple steps
Infrequent production

Patient-centric vision demands effective collaboration among all disciplines in an integrated healthcare delivery system. Information systems, networks, communications interfaces, links, diagnostic and therapeutic technologies must be iteratively reengineered through process improvement initiatives (QM, BPR, Six Sigma) in order to deliver and sustain delivery of seamless effective patient care.

> Lean thinking is a determination of value that distinguishes value-added steps from non–value-added steps, then eliminating waste.

To maximize value and eliminate waste in health care, leaders must first evaluate processes by identifying and specifying value for every step in care delivery processes (value streams in Lean language). Then individuals or teams must be tasked with responsibility to eliminate non–value-added steps and make value flow from beginning to end. Lean principles have a dramatic effect on productivity, cost, and quality. When applied rigorously throughout an entire IDS, "pull" defines the needs of patients and other customers. The alternative of "pull" principles is unproductive and usually outdated "push" processes which do not add any value.

Table 13.2 highlights dramatic results achieved in other industries as Lean thinking and principles were applied. There is no reason that similar results will not be realized in health care. Implementing Lean thinking requires a change in management priorities and resourced initiatives throughout entire organizations. Such refocused priorities will incorporate disruptive technologies that are traumatic by design and expectedly difficult. Strong commitment and inspiring leadership from senior leaders is essential to success in these challenging endeavors. Leaders must be vocal and visible champions of Lean management by creating an environment where failure is permissible and goals encourage "leaps of faith." A senior management team that is aligned in vision and understanding of Lean strategies is a perquisite foundation for "going Lean."

A "Lean culture" is a necessary foundation upon which patient-centered and seamless digitized processes can be transformed with lean tools and techniques. Lean organization culture differs from a traditional culture in other service industries. Health care need not be an exception.

Table 13.3 compares these cultural transformational differences.

> An organization's culture is a set of values and beliefs that cause staff to behave in certain ways. When all staff members behave in that way and achieve expected results, values and beliefs are reinforced. This self-reinforcing cycle creates and sustains organizational culture.

Lean culture requires new behaviors in smaller, "right-sized" teams of workers or technologies in "cells." Strong situational leadership must augment team approaches to achieve more "right now" real-time action, rather than traditional, less effective work batching.

TABLE 13.2   Impact of Lean Principles on Other Industries

Direct labor/productivity improved	45–75%
Cost reduced	25–55%
Throughput/flow increased	60–90%
Quality improved or defects reduced	50–90%
Inventory reduced	60–90%
Space requirements reduced	35–50%
Lead time reduced	50–90%

TABLE 13.3   Traditional Versus Lean Cultures

Traditional Culture	Lean Culture
Silo functions	Interdisciplinary teams
Managers directing	Managers teaching and enabling
Benchmarking to justify "just as good"	Seeking performance without waste
Blaming people	Identifying and addressing root cause
Rewarding individuals	Recognizing team successes
Considering suppliers enemies	Collaborating with supplier as ally
Guarding information	Sharing information
Lowering cost by increasing volume	Removing waste to lower cost
Internal focus	Patient and customer focus
Driven by experts	Driven by process

The IHI recommends that many management and operations tools that have been developed and refined in other industries be successfully applied in healthcare process and quality improvement. Lean principles reduce or eliminate wasted time, resources, and energy in health care. Lean approaches create systems, applications, and processes that are integrated, inter-operative, efficient, and effectively responsive to patient requirements expectations.

SUMMARY

This chapter introduced and explained Lean enterprise terminology, tools, techniques, and concepts by describing how Lean principles and approaches are applicable in healthcare provider organizations.

Fundamental concepts and content focused on

- Lean enterprise metrics
- Strategies, tools, and principles to increase efficiency, decrease waste, and improve quality
- VSM and visual management
- Error-proofing and standardizing operations
- Push versus pull systems and takt time

CHAPTER QUESTIONS

These questions reinforce student understanding, learning, and retention while stimulating class discussion:

1. Outline expectations of implementing Lean strategies in healthcare organizations based on experiences in other industries.
2. Explain how Lean strategies and QM are related as well as how they are associated with J. Edward Deming and Toyota.
3. Summarize results of Lean strategy implementation at Virginia Mason Medical Center.
4. Explain the most significant change to emergency treatment process as depicted in Figure 13.2.
5. Outline the most common causes of human error and how they differ from process errors.

ADDITIONAL RESOURCES

These references are recommended for additional reading and more comprehensive content beyond the scope of this book.

Coile, Jr., R. (2002). The Paperless Hospital: Healthcare in a Digital Age. Chicago: Health Administration Press.

Deming, E. Quality and Statistical Process Control. Cambridge, MA: MIT Center for Advanced Engineering Study.

Goldsmith, J. (2003). Digital Medicine Implications for Healthcare Leaders. Chicago: Health Administration Press.

Larson, J. (2001). Management Engineering. Chicago: Healthcare Information and Management Systems Society.

Longest, Jr., B., Rakich, J., Darr, K. (2004). Managing Health Services Organizations and Systems. Baltimore, MD: Health Professions Press.

Tufte, E. (1990).Visual Explanations. Cheshire, CT: Graphics Press.

Tufte, E. (1997). Envisioning Information. Cheshire, CT: Graphics Press.

Tufte, E. (1997). The Visual Display of Information. Cheshire, CT: Graphics Press.

CHAPTER 14

Telemedicine and Clinical Informatics

This chapter introduces telemedicine and clinical informatics, focusing on these concepts:

- Definitions and fundamentals of informatics, e-medicine, and telemedicine
- E-health applications
- Health decision support systems
- Data warehousing (DW) and data mining (DM)

Informatics embodies an ever-expanding set of specialized IT applications of care delivery processes, decision support, and research, including a variety of IT systems and applications and capabilities. Clinical informatics incorporates and analyzes opportunities and impacts associated with increasingly interoperable, interdependent applications. For example:

- Databases and DM derived from insurance claims processing
- Applications enabling providers to diagnose and treat patients and deliver ongoing care with significantly improved quality, efficiency, effectiveness, and safety without limitation of location
- Effective remote monitoring of increasingly patient-centric care delivery
- Innovative new therapies throughout and beyond traditional provider networks
- Empowered providers to remotely deliver and monitor treatments and therapy, as well as ever increasing variety of services directly to independently living patients, enabling some to remain in the community and "age in place."

184

Health informatics and telemedicine emphasize clinical and biomedical applications of e-health technologies.

As healthcare professionals have become more computer-literate and have demonstrated enhanced multidisciplinary competencies, medicine, patient-centric care delivery, and IT are increasingly interoperable, interdependent, and essentially inseparable.

Increasingly more user-friendly, powerful, and faster IT empowers healthcare professionals in all medical research and patient-centric care delivery venues to provide advanced levels of specialized care that improves life-sustaining and life-saving delivery capabilities.

As an example, this case study demonstrates savings from improved quality of care and reduced cost. More than 150 hospitals are participating in a novel service that enables "virtual intensive care expertise and real-time supplemental support."

Remote monitoring and clinical decision-support technology connects expert treatment by critical care nurses and attending physicians with specialized skills of intensivists. These specialists are in high demand, expensive and are difficult to employ.

CASE STUDY

This model is an "e-ICU" program developed in response to economic barriers experienced by hospitals in staffing intensive care units (ICUs) with specially trained nurses and intensivists. Intensivists are board-certified physicians specializing in care to patients in an ICU. Technology of the type described in this case study requires real-time integration of audio-wave files, visual images, and clinical data.

A 2007 study by the Leapfrog Group, a think tank that monitors and benchmarks healthcare effectiveness and innovation, revealed that few of America's ICUs had full-time access to a critical care physician. Without this level of specialized physician support, hospital deaths were unacceptably higher than expected.

Despite this troublesome national trend, a small group of providers implemented an innovative solution to this critical care delivery problem. A 2004 analysis of this pioneering technology reported that:

- A 27% reduction in severity-adjusted hospital ICU mortality rates among monitored ICU patients because 20% of these patients were more successfully treated than national benchmarks

- A 17% reduction in ICU length of stay
- More than $2,000 cost-savings per patient stay

More than 150 hospitals use these always-on, real-time, ICU monitoring and decision-support capabilities for more than 4,000 beds in more than 300 ICUs. A recent survey of ICU nurses working in ICUs using this approach concluded that nurses were supportive of this capability. These ICUs enjoyed higher nursing retention rates in these ICUs than in units not using this application. ICU nurses appreciated an expert resource available at any time for questions or consultations. They reported feeling reassured that this support network provided a "second opinion" safety net.

This application augments bedside teams with additional resources to monitor patients. An additional "expert" monitoring layer more closely observes patients, rapidly identifies patient conditions if they begin to deteriorate, and directs appropriate real-time intervention. "Virtual intensivists" at a remote command center continually monitor and evaluate subtle changes in patient status, such as slight dips in blood oxygenation or hemoglobin levels, dilated pupils, and so on. Cameras, videoconferencing systems, and special software operate at each patient's bedside, feeding critical data to an on-duty clinician at the virtual command center. These virtual intensivists alert physicians and nurses in the ICU to administer necessary intervention as appropriate.

Initial pilot tests of this system demonstrated improved quality of care for critically ill patients and reduced patient care costs with reduced ICU lengths of stay. Project team leaders implementing this system in each participating hospital used strategies to ensure that this virtual support function was fully integrated and that everyone worked well as an effective virtual team.

Applications of this type require rapid technologic advances that enable systems to support rather than impede care delivery via IT-driven digital process transformation. As a society, America is now enjoying that nexus of hardware advance and software utility. For example, as of this writing, Moore's Law has once more been demonstrated. (Microchip power and processing speed continues to advance every 18 months with significantly more transistors per microchip.) More transistors on a microchip enable microchip manufacturers to produce commercial versions of denser multi-core processors using a 30 nm process with hafnium-based high-dielectric and metal gates to decrease current leakage and yield faster, more energy-efficient microchips. These new materials demonstrated a non-silicon solution resolves manufacturing problems encountered with silicon chips as the traditional process shrank below the 65 nm threshold.

Healthcare informatics is both an art and science of innovative information and IT technology to discover historically unrecognized relationships that enable optimal decision-making. Informatics is more than IT, incorporating a rationale for how and why clinicians need, acquire, and use information.

Core competencies for "informaticians" are evolving but minimally include capabilities such as

- Demonstrating multi-disciplinary and domain-specific knowledge
- Understanding information systems theory, including fundamental logic and limited fourth- and fifth-generation language programming skills
- Communicating and collaborating with multi-disciplinary colleagues in key areas (researchers, clinical applications developers, decision-support systems users, as well as other professionals in evaluative and analytic sciences).

A troublesome "occupational liability" associated with informatics is that rapidly advancing IT and medical science often render discipline-specific expertise and "trendy" technologic competencies obsolete. An optimal blend of informatics and discipline-specific knowledge is ambiguous about the degree to which principles of informatics are inherently abstracted and principles that are linked to discipline-specific applications.

E-medicine evolved during the last quarter century, initially relying on cumbersome, slow, low-cost telephone technology. Limited funding delayed significant advances until health computing and networking technologies were commonplace. Interest has expanded in a variety of settings, such as e-medicine, administrative, clinical, e-commerce, e-health, e-clinical decision support, and expert systems. Additionally, e-nursing support systems, e-prescribing, and other e-health applications, such as e-home care systems, intelligent medical information systems, and health decision support systems (HDSS), have become commonplace.

Clinical informaticians expect to replicate and enhance cognitive processes of clinicians. Researchers want to add intelligence to information systems and, by extension, to remote medical diagnostic systems. These systems demonstrate multi-disciplinary and domain-specific knowledge that enables communication and collaboration with colleagues in key areas.

EVOLVING PERSPECTIVES

With these new technologies and substantial investments during the last decade, issues of privacy and security and related processes became necessary to protect healthcare information from a variety of threats. IT professionals, researchers, providers, and other businesses rapidly focused on network and Internet connectivity. Internet applications quickly evolved from military and academic origins with rapid widespread discovery and proliferation of e-mail as convenient, but insecure communications technology. E-commerce and e-business concepts began revolutionizing business process redesign, process automation, and quality improvement as society experienced, enjoyed and became increasingly proficient in emerging Internet technologies.

Ubiquitous, exponential growth of these constantly evolving "disruptive technologies" beneficially extend e-technologies in many patient-centric delivery venues. Specifically targeted and uniquely healthcare-oriented applications include:

- Intranets
- Extranets
- Virtual public and private networks
- E-business networks
- Web-based businesses
- Community networks and learning communities

Web-based development services and health maintenance organizations expanded into a variety of e-health perspectives, domains, technologies, and applications. In this context, revolutionary diffusion of IT-driven e-health tools, is a paradigm shift from traditional physician and clinician-centered delivery applications to a consumer-driven patient-centric system. E-health systems focus on patients rather than on caregivers. That said, supporting processes require radical reengineering and redesign to ensure that this potential is realized. E-health applications are commonly used by patients in progressive health maintenance organizations and health plans to connect with member physicians as required, whenever and wherever a need arises. Patient and physician relationships are no longer limited by time and space.

IT has enabled convenient switching of providers when a patient's expectation of service or product quality or level of health knowledge and expertise of a provider, health maintenance organization, or health plan is not met. Accelerated and consistent flow of e-health data, information, knowledge, and wisdom enables patients to be more assertive and empowered in more challenging roles. Patients now have ready access to creditable world-class information sources.

Patients are educating themselves in

- Cost-effective evidence-based medical practices and integrative gene-based medicine
- Alternative and complementary clinical modalities
- Health-promoting life-styles, activities, and behaviors

These actions and changes in e-patient and e-consumer behaviors demand new and creative forms of consumer-driven, patient-centric, health information therapies.

INFORMATICS APPLICATIONS

E-health and applications exist in domains with similar dimensions and integration characteristics. Applications and technologies integrated or interoperable *within* an organization are defined as internally integrated.

Examples of these highly integrated applications include

- Virtual patient records (VPRs)
- Document management
- Geographic information systems (GIS)
- Health decision-support systems
- Executive information systems (EIS/DW/DM)

Alternatively, other applications exhibit a high degree of external integration (networks, systems, applications, and associated technologic interfaces) with other providers, payers, governmental, or other agency computer systems that are external to healthcare provider organization:

- Telecommunications
- Wireless networks
- Application service providers
- Virtual private networks
- Community health information networks (CHINs)
- Internet, intranets, and extranets
- Health informatics
- Telemedicine or e-medicine

VPR technology houses uniquely identifiable information about an individual patient from various isolated sources. Diversified data are encoded in different formats for use with different platforms and converted for use on a common virtual platform.

This concept is not creating a massive traditional database, but rather to develop a common inter-operative infrastructure, enabling component interaction and operation as an open system. This approach supports conversion and transmission of media-rich medical data from multiple distributed sources supporting multiple users.

Health informatics and telemedicine emphasize clinical and biomedical applications of e-health technologies.

Tele-Med, a collaborative VPR prototype project created by researchers at Los Alamos National Laboratory and physicians from the National Jewish Medical and Research Center in Denver, supports real-time interactive uses of media-rich graphic patient records among multiple users at multiple sites.

VPR technologies are ideal for telemedicine, For example, online clinical and financial data that is instantaneously available with document management technology (**DM**). Document management (DM) applications include document imaging, workflow optimization, electronic form processing, off-line mass data storage, and other evolving technologies. Many hospitals and health organizations use document management technology to handle otherwise paper-intensive processes required to collect and file patient information. For example, wireless notebook computers and customized software enable nurses to rapidly and accurately update all patient and insurance records electronically instead of handwriting and later transcribing documents and forms between visits to patients. This technology enables physicians and nurses to deliver more, higher quality, safer and affordable care.

GIS applications are powerful tools for collecting, recording, storing, analyzing, and displaying spatial data sets. GIS use spatial data, such as digitized maps displaying a combination of text, graphics, icons, and symbols on multidimensional maps. GIS technology is used for digital mapping. For example, identifying and treating an epidemic (HIV infection among a subpopulation across various counties in a state). Specific population groups are targeted for intervention with this knowledge.

An HDSS bundles analytic modeling and network communications to support group decision-making processes (strategic thinking, problem formulation, and generation of goal-seeking solutions). HDSS reduce both the cognitive burden and the mental effort associated with group meetings. This technology also has the potential to increase the efficiency, effectiveness, and productivity of group interactions through asynchronous board meetings, online forums, or special group meetings. Clinicians and executives share information without constraint of time and distance.

In the context of any health provider organization, an EIS collects, filters, and extracts a broad range of current and historical e-health–related information from multiple applications and across external and internal data sources. These applications provide executives with necessary information to identify key problems and strategic opportunities. A common EIS application is long-distance strategic planning sessions to determine and prioritize the challenges of various business strategies. One popular feature is the ability of an EIS to narrow or expand information from one level to another, enabling executives to conveniently retrieve answers to special or ad-hoc queries. For example, a decision support system that allows a health manager to know who and why a group of people are frequent users of the organization's emergency services enables implementation of policies to prevent resource abuse or misuse.

Another important feature is the ease with which EIS technology is integrated with other technologies, such as GIS and HDSS.

DW is a contemporary architecture for integrated information management that functions as a source of aggregated, organized, and formatted data. Data in a data warehouse are designed to support management decision-making and strategic planning. By increasing data analysis and processing power, a provider can develop new and more complex e-health technologies.

Common applications of an e-health DW include automatically collecting vast amounts of linked data from diverse sources for use in DM techniques.

DM techniques explore data to identify trends and patterns. DM tools include artificial intelligence, neural e-health networks, case-based reasoning, statistical methods, genetic algorithms, and explanation-based reasoning. Discovery of best practices is achieved by comparing and contrasting physician practice patterns. Analyses of different treatment protocols for specific patient case mixes is one complementary benefit of applying both DW and DM technologies. Human genome mapping to provide treatments for various challenging ailments is an example.

This case study is an example of a statewide resource in which this author participated in early policymaking. Developing and formulating protocol from a hospital CIO perspective was advantageous. As a member of the first advisory board chartered, this author was uniquely qualified to ensure that end-user, real-world concerns were addressed during development and implementation of legislated regulations and mandates.

CASE STUDY

An independent agency, The Pennsylvania Health Care Cost Containment Council (PHC4), was established by a Pennsylvania statute in 1986 to address accelerating healthcare costs.

Early strategies focused on this mandated objective to contain costs and benchmark healthcare quality and stimulate competition:

- Publishing comparative information about the most efficient and effective healthcare providers for employers, business coalitions, individual consumers and other group purchasers of health services

- Providing database access to information that is collected, aggregated, and analyzed by mandate to identify opportunities to contain costs and improve the quality of care delivery
- Collecting, analyzing, and publishing quarterly and annual reports for employers, business coalitions, and patients about benchmarked healthcare cost and quality delivered by Pennsylvania providers
- Studying access issues, such as access to care by uninsured Pennsylvanians
- Proposing and reviewing mandated health insurance benefits by legislative and executive branches of state government

Each year PHC4 collects more than 4 million inpatient hospital discharge and outpatient procedure records from Pennsylvania hospitals and freestanding ambulatory surgery centers. This information is transmitted in HIPAA-compliant formats each quarter by each provider. This data set includes detailed data verified by each provider (benchmarked care quality, provider hospital charge, cost and treatment information, as well as other financial data).

PHC4 shares these data through free public reports. Since 1986 PHC4 has published hundreds of reports about Pennsylvania healthcare delivery efficiency, effectiveness, quality, and cost. These reports are widely distributed and are accessible through PHC4's website (www.phc4.org) and in public libraries throughout Pennsylvania.

PHC4 has produced thousands of customized reports and data sets as required by legislation or upon request from providers, policymakers, researchers, insurers, and other group purchasers of healthcare services.

PHC4 was one of the first such agencies chartered. Similar organizations have been mandated on a state-by-state basis.

These organizations and applications have a high degree of external integration, such as e-health networking technologies. These applications speed up large-scale exchange of media-rich health information from one point to another on a network. These network architectures are configured as

- Hub-and-wheel communication
- Open systems
- Internet-based, HIPAA-compliant, secure electronic data interchange
- Extranets or intranets
- Groupware applications

These organizations are often sponsored by leaders of emerging technologies. Even though they may be aggressive competitors in the commercial healthcare IT marketplace, these sponsors facilitate state and regional technology deployment by developing and sustaining collaborative workgroups. The North Carolina Communication and Healthcare Communication Alliance and e-PA, the e-Pennsylvania Alliance, are two examples of this type of regional collaboration.

A CHIN is a network that links healthcare stakeholders throughout a community or region. Such an integrated collection of telecommunication and networking capabilities is an infrastructure to enable communication with patients and clinical and financial information exchange among and between multiple providers, payers, employers, pharmacies, and regional healthcare organizations. An effective CHIN requires practical implementation of computerized patient record systems within each community, or a broader regional, statewide and national level.

CHIN technology is an interactive research and communication tool for medical professionals and healthcare consumers searching for health-related information and knowledge. Intranets and extranets extend this concept by using the Internet as an inexpensive, reliable, and comprehensive web of global networks. These networks use standardized hardware and software infrastructure to build, manage, sustain, expand, enhance, browse, and search websites.

Unlike the Internet, these virtual networks may be private and protected by security software (firewalls) to keep unauthorized users from gaining access.

An intranet supports Internet-based services only for an organization's staff or members. Extranets extend network access privileges to certain partners with access to selected areas inside a private virtual network, thereby creating a secure customer or vendor network.

Representative applications of these concepts include:

- An integrated Internet, intranet, and extranet used in digitally transformed healthcare delivery venues enable "e-users" (patients, physicians, and other healthcare professionals) to access online insurance data and required clinical service information.
- Electronic filing of insurance benefits, claims, and payment remittances via extranets dramatically reduces organizational overhead and labor costs while increasing information accessibility by patients and providers. These capabilities enable administrative insight into medical best practice and healthcare delivery trends.

Intranets and extranets provide privacy, security and accuracy of transactions by using information encryption and transmission over secure lines to ensure confidentiality. Although intranets share internal data within an organization, the Internet and extranets connect selected users from outside an organization to public information.

From a more technological and terminology intensive perspective, e-HDSS, e-clinical decision support systems, and e-expert decision support systems assist physicians and other medical specialists in diagnosis, therapeutic, and related aspects of care delivery.

One example of an e-clinical decision support system is an interactive system that enables a clinician or patient to enter personal health data to understand and evaluate various options related to a surgical intervention.

HDSS is a generic term used among administration staff, whereas e-clinical decision support system denote a clinical focus and may be systems used by health providers. In contrast, an e-expert decision support system may be a discipline-specific application for specialists. Common applications include:

- Monitor patient heart rates and alert care providers when abnormal rates are detected
- Guide prescribing physicians and pharmacists as alerts for potentially adverse drug interactions
- Educate patients on preventive health care and health-promoting activities
- Perform virtual diagnosis of disease and disorders

Tele-radiology has been widely used to scan digitized patient images, store images electronically, and share images with health providers at geographically distant sites.

Similar e-medicine applications include:

- Pathology, surgery, and cardiac catheterization consultations
- Clinical robotics
- Virtual reality learning, videoconferencing, or online medical education
- Tele-care

Anticipated exponential growth potential, critical aspects of e-health systems must include planning a strategic vision, developing business strategy, and managing technology innovation that aligns senior management goals with changing needs of e-health markets. Planners of these applications must proactively identify e-consumer needs and e-business requirements, apply systems and decision theory, embrace e-marketing and virtual network management concepts as well as support DM and DM mining. These traditional business and system planning applications reflect an acknowledgment that e-health data, information, and knowledge are shared resources and that acceptance of any e-health business model requires collaboration and consensus-building of e-health participating professionals, payers, and consumers.

System and scenario planning are techniques used to evaluate competing futures, envision strategies, and develop and test against each possible future. These approaches generate an e-technology vision that reflects scenario results and incorporates an assessment of system capabilities and limitations.

Successful e-health system planning requires management of the entire technologic infrastructure and information processing capacity of virtual business systems. Senior management must embrace these visionary concepts to ensure that information resources and e-technology are best adapted to meet patient and care provider needs. Transaction protocols and standards must be integrated into existing administrative procedures and e-technologies with legacy systems and new innovative applications in a virtual network infrastructure.

Administrative issues include policies and procedures that reinforce network standards for privacy, security, and confidentiality of virtual patient and e-patient records as well as legal and ethical considerations regarding data collected, analyzed, and distributed electronically. Legacy system implementation and evaluation deficits were historically associated with inferior design or poor interface configuration. Effective and efficient interfaces are significant and must be emphasized because patients, providers, administrative users, and e-consumers now commonly conduct businesses through these interfaces, rather than by face-to-face interaction.

E-health system implementation and evaluation challenges are functional requirements. They include integration of planning, control, and improvement processes, safe, secure, well-managed, patient-centric care in a quality-focused e-healthcare environment. These e-health system components require further integration of network technology, operations management, organizational collaboration, and user interface technology management that builds an efficient IDS-wide system infrastructure. Sustained integration of these electronically gathered data, aggregated information, models, and knowledge into effectively designed applications are critical resource utilization challenges. These implementation challenges require project management (as explained in Chapter 7), as well as comprehensive program evaluation.

E-health system implementation and evaluation must incorporate organizational and environmental changes and system modifications:

- E-networking infrastructure
- Competence requirement for e-workers
- Efficient information flow and effective clinical and administrative practice and processes
- Belief systems, life-styles, ethics, and behaviors of staff and patients

Senior leadership must ensure that clinicians and other users gain, retain, and sustain critical knowledge, skills, and aptitudes to address these changes (staffing, training, and educational considerations). Attracting and retaining talented technical staff requires aggressive recruitment and retention programs, staff training, development and deployment of e-learning opportunities, and strategies to encourage shared knowledge, intelligence, and expertise.

E-health incorporates improved and increased capabilities for individual clinicians, system users, and patients via virtual alliances, workgroups, management, interactions, networking and collaborative decision-making. For example, a VPR that is accessible by multiple care providers integrates patient history, diagnostics, treatments and therapeutic information from various disciplines for each patient. E-health system impacts will eventually extend to and through every aspect of healthcare delivery at both a community and societal level.

Technology advance has already had significant impacts in these early years of the 21st century, for example:

- Telecommuting and virtual work by e-health workers
- Innovative tools, techniques, applications, and opportunities for seniors and disabled workers (automated support technology and robotics to reduce risk of injury for workers in hazardous environments)
- Increased potential for abuse and misuse of these powerful resources, tools, and techniques
- Improved purchasing of healthcare options, including new modalities of care with enhanced capabilities to reach distant consumers and otherwise underserved populations

SUMMARY

Early benefits are radically impacting medical practice, care delivery, as well as each patient's quality of life. As the pace and intensity of these "disruptive technologies" accelerate, healthcare providers and individual healthcare workers are being driven to deliver and practice within this e-health model. Rapidly changing demographics and reimbursement incentives are driving the healthcare delivery industry along this e-health pathway with significant career and life-style impacts.

This chapter introduced terminology, techniques, and clinical informatics concepts and outlined implications for healthcare providers.

Key concepts included:

- Definitions and current status of informatics, e-medicine, and telemedicine DW and DM
- E-health applications
- HDSS

CHAPTER QUESTIONS

These questions reinforce student understanding, learning, and retention while stimulating class discussion:

1. Explain how informatics and telemedicine are related.
2. What is data warehousing?
3. How is data mining accomplished?
4. Is PHC4 both a data warehouse and a decision-support system? Explain.

ADDITIONAL RESOURCES

These references are recommended for additional reading and more comprehensive content beyond the scope of this book.

Griffith, J., White, K. (2002). The Well-Managed Healthcare Organization. Chicago: Health Administration Press.

Longest, Jr., B., Rakich, J., Darr, K. (2004). Managing Health Services Organizations and Systems. Baltimore, MD: Health Professions Press.

Nelson, R. (1999). Tele-health: Changing healthcare in the twenty-first century. Journal of Health Information Management, 13(4).

Newell, L. (2000). Beyond year 2000: Innovative solutions for the evolving healthcare information management environment. Journal of Health Information Management, 14(1).

Tufte, E. (1990).Visual Explanations. Cheshire, CT: Graphics Press.

Tufte, E. (1997). Envisioning Information. Cheshire, CT: Graphics Press.

Tufte, E. (1997). The Visual Display of Information. Cheshire, CT: Graphics Press.

CHAPTER 15

Emerging Technologies

This chapter introduces emerging technologies as envisioned by healthcare futurists and IT experts to be in widespread use within this decade.

These "disruptive technologies" are having significant impact on all providers. More robust capabilities must address escalating societal demands for radically improved, higher quality, lower cost, and more patient-centric healthcare delivery processes. Effective digital transformation of healthcare delivery processes requires the application of these technologies in a well-planned, disciplined, and adequately funded manner.

Key concepts include

- National healthcare information infrastructure (NHII)
- Digital systems continuum
- Clinical technology opportunities and challenges
- A digital health community (DHC)
- Paradigm shifts or innovative conceptual constructs
- Multifaceted technologies

An important emerging technology is the planning and implementing of an NHII. As this NHII becomes fully operational, providers will be able to provide care for patients in a multitude of safer and innovative ways. For example, fewer patients will require hospital admission as providers and other members of the healthcare team monitor and care for them at home.

President G. W. Bush has challenged America to implement a fully automated electronic medical records (EMRs) by 2014. These significant objectives and key components are included in this daunting endeavor:

- Establish government-wide health IT governance council
- Identify portfolio of 24 target domains for data and messaging standards
- Partner with 23 federal agencies/departments who use health data to build adopted standards into their health IT architecture
- Adopt messaging and terminology standards for 20 domains, yielding 11 sets of standards to be used in federal IT architectures
- Adopt domains that are standards ready or mature enough to produce follow-up recommendations
- Establish, fund, host, and sustain regular meetings with industry leaders to prevent major incompatibilities in partnership with the National Committee on Vital and Health Statistics
- Define management role changes for this initiative's merger into a federal health architecture
- Incorporate consolidated health informatics goals into the federal health architecture and activities coordinated through the Office of the National Coordinator for Health Information Technology (http://www.hhs.gov/healthit/)
- Present consolidated health informatics standards to the Health Information Technology Standards Panel and the American Health Information Community that incorporate national health interoperability standards that are compatible with all components to yield a truly harmonized process

Additionally President Bush envisions America to sponsor, support, and enable development of an operating DHC that is compatible with countries that are already engaged in planning an NHII. Although there are differences in approach in each country, common attributes include these key components of traditional health information management:

- individual health records are created with each patient possessing or with access to his or her own personal health record.
- patient health record including an individual's health and medication history, acute and chronic health conditions, history, and health insurance, other reimbursement information.
- provider access and update compatibility for these data in individual patient health records with physicians' notes and other relevant clinical information.
- provider access to tools such as digital prescription applications that update individual health records, generate an order to provide requested products and services to manage national health, identify costs, conduct research, etc.
- support for public health agencies, epidemiologists, and other population health analysts to accumulate, aggregate, analyze, and report population health data, trends, or patterns.

NHII STATUS AND CURRENT STRATEGY

These NHII concepts are being developed in the United States as an NHIN, with oversight through the Office of the National Coordinator for Health Information Technology. America's NHIN is envisioned as an information and knowledge-sharing network that incorporates interoperable technologies and standards but is not a central database of patient records.

Current status of major nation-wide federal government-driven projects is best reflected in 2008 executive summaries of published reports reflecting nationally adopted standards:

- Medications: Summary Report including Special Populations and Drug Classifications
- Medications: Structured Product Labeling Sections
- Medications: Drug Product
- Medications: Package
- Medications: Active Ingredients
- Medications: Clinical Drug
- Medications: Manufactured Dosage Form
- Anatomy
- Billing/Financial
- Chemicals
- Clinical Encounters
- Diagnosis and Problem Lists
- Genes and Proteins
- Immunizations
- Interventions & Procedures, Laboratory Test Order Names
- Interventions and Procedures, Non-Laboratory
- Laboratory Result Contents
- Nursing
- Text Based Reports
- Units

Recognizing the dynamic nature of such a list, the current status of these projects and the overall initiative can be reviewed at anytime at this website: http://www .hhs.gov/healthit/. This initiative involves many healthcare-related stakeholders, for example, individual and organizational providers, consumers (patient representatives), private and governmental agencies, professional organizations, and payers.

Unless Electronic Health Record (EHR) systems communicate, they are simply islands of data where patient information does not flow seamlessly from one clinical setting to the next. Without clinicians' ability to exchange information with one another electronically, whether across town or across the country, patients' information may not be readily available when and where as needed. To remedy this currently unacceptable state, an interoperable system based on a common architecture is being developed. Patient records will be available electronically virtually anywhere. Three fundamental strategies are required to address these specifications.

The first strategy is to foster regional collaboration among healthcare entities so that a patient's information is securely stored in a local community database and is electronically accessible to all authorized clinicians involved with providing care in that community. A limited number of regional initiatives exist today. Because their approaches to data-sharing vary, they cannot communicate patient information outside their own system. As momentum builds and more collaborative regional health information organizations (RHIOs) are formed, a common approach will develop and will support an overall goal of healthcare data exchange.

A second strategy in this very broadly scoped initiative is to include the government in the formation of RHIOs. These local RHIOs must use a common set of standards to communicate with one another. Interconnecting each RHIO requires an infrastructure, known as an NHIN, to facilitate interoperability among RHIOs. Each standard enables authorized providers to access medical information flow any time anywhere. This strategy revolutionizes health care industry-wide by making information more patient and consumer centric. DHHS proposed convening a private sector consortium to plan, develop, and operate the NHIN and published a Request for Information for public sector input into the design and operation of the NHIN.

A third strategy confirms the federal government's commitment to funding, leading, and mandating use of common standards and architecture to achieve a result similar to plans in the private sector. RHIO implementations are underway as a bottom-up rather than a top-down adoption strategy. As regional information interchange is demonstrated, "lessons learned" and more "hands-on experience" will mold the NHII concept by driving a comprehensive nation-wide implementation. As with all politics, health care is local and regional, with most benefits experienced at community and regional provider levels.

Interest in the NHII concept is growing regionally, nationally, and globally. As successes are demonstrated, regions, states, and countries are learning from each other. These data standard recommendations are being built to incorporate earlier collaborations with:

- Office of the National Coordinator
- Consolidated Health Informatics Initiative
- Markle Foundation
- Certification Commission for Healthcare Information Technology

- Health Information and Management Systems Society
- Health Level Seven
- California HealthCare Foundation, especially Interoperability and Connectivity Standards

A digitally transformed community hospital is the key nexus on a continuum as healthcare delivery organizations incrementally automate their core processes. Rather than a final goal, each digitalized provider is another milestone on a path to becoming another pioneering organization that enjoys increasingly effective capabilities. These emerging technologies benefit all patients and providers. As an organizational driver to an ever-evolving goal, each community hospital is being rapidly and cost-efficiently transformed as a digital, fully automated, highly responsive organization that melds into a seamless, comprehensive, patient-centric DHC.

Such a DHC will evolve and be fully achieved over time with deliberate incremental automation and interconnectivity between and among digital healthcare providers in a locale. From a patient's perspective, although hospitals are very important they do not provide all care, especially for chronic conditions. Hospitals must champion a smooth and seamless integration (not an isolated island of disjointed care processes) among and between other provider organizations delivering care to each individual patient. Potential opportunities for connectivity and interoperability result in improved healthcare processes with attending and referring physicians, payers, reference laboratories, tertiary care centers, rehabilitation centers, and other participants in healthcare delivery. More health care occurs in communities and not primarily in hospitals. A critical healthcare industry challenge is to define and integrate this current complex array of misaligned incentives and legislative barriers that have historically impeded progress toward more productive and more effective information sharing. This lack of sharing reflects traditional provincial aspects of healthcare delivery that have been recognized but not addressed.

At one end of this dynamic continuum of increasing digitization, current healthcare providers are organizations that are all too reliant on manual and paper-based processes within poorly interfaced silos of care. At the other end of this continuum are digitally transformed communities of organizations functioning as essentially efficient and effectively paper-free components of a patient-centric system of healthcare delivery. Each component of this "ideal system" must embrace and use state-of-the-art IT to ensure that all relevant information is consistently accessible any time and anywhere within a global DHC.

A core component of this DHC is a digital hospital requiring transformation and integration of many processes, applications, and other components. This transformation is and will continue to be a formidable challenge.

Some core components of each digital hospital are still at a "proof of concept" stage. Initially, an essential foundation of key infrastructure is broadly adopted with well-defined standards and technologies. IT architecture is integrated in a strategic framework that reflects tactical deployment of automated solutions. This process is well underway.

Conceptual breakthroughs are not new, with many of these breakthroughs more than a half century old (El Camino Hospital circa 1965). Current technologies (high-speed networks, WANs, low cost computers, and fifth-generation software) are available. These tools, techniques, technologies, and other transformation enablers provide an essential critical mass to "move forward smartly" on in a comprehensive and pervasive fast track.

Expected benefits from any significant IT investment will only be realized when senior leadership drives genuine organization-wide focus on deep ubiquitous process redesign.

Digital initiatives must move beyond just implementing a paperless or digital information system. Incremental value in each component's investment must reflect sufficient critical mass and be scaled large enough to be constructively disruptive, yet ultimately demonstrate organization-wide process-driven transformation.

PICTURE ARCHIVING AND COMMUNICATION SYSTEMS (PACS)

A traditional implementation of a departmental PACS solution is an imaging application enabling digital processing of radiological imaging between scanners, radiologists in a reading room, requesting physician, and other authorized providers. Implementation of PACS in imaging departments during the last decade have demonstrated significantly improved workflow while reducing clinical and administrative workload by:

- Eliminating film-produced images, thus permitting entire clinical processes to be redesigned so that images are available virtually anywhere at any time
- Rapid and more accurate diagnostic decisions have been achieved and have enabled digital transformation of diagnostic pathways. These obviously beneficial capabilities are leveraging initial investments to generate comparable benefits throughout the entire enterprise

When PACS is used to automate workflow as a comprehensive enterprise-wide solution rather than exclusively as a departmental application, opportunity for task consolidation and elimination results in additional benefits from an initial "departmental" investment.

Increasing numbers of providers are demonstrating innovative aspects and applications of PACS as an effective driver for core process transformation. Following are examples of PACS enabling and enhancing real-time communication beyond radiology and cardiology imaging:

- Automation of nursing medication administration and pharmacy communication and processing
- Physician office integration to support computerized physician order entry (CPOE)
- More clinical knowledge management
- Community outreach initiatives targeting greater patient engagement

A fully implemented PACS serves as an essential foundation and infrastructure upon which a comprehensive EMR can evolve. Experience in earlier adopter organizations has shown that a functional EMR is an essential prerequisite for healthcare providers to realize benefits achieved with a successful CPOE installation. Effective clinical knowledge management is almost impossible without CPOE. If nursing and pharmacy process automation are not embedded in an organization's operations, CPOE is unlikely to succeed. A well-planned and IT strategy depends on incremental and parallel deployment of these key components, applications, and systems.

Technology interdependence and interoperability between and among key processes are more daunting challenges without interoperability, integration, and interdependency that demands real-time or need real-time resolution (formulary or order set development and maintenance).

CLINICAL TECHNOLOGY CHALLENGES

Legacy clinical information systems have improved efficiency and quality of care within individual departments, but not among departments. More challenging integration and inter-operative capabilities must be realized before clinicians can truly deliver patient-centric care without paper-bound distraction. Unless such critical mass of IT transformation, clinicians will continue to unproductively search for reports or test results, illegibly ordering error-prone, unsafe care.

The terms *electronic medical, patient,* and *health records* have been used interchangeably throughout this text. However, in the context of a DHC evolution, terms reflect different record content and degree of difficulty to digitize. In this context, an EMR is a database of patient data that is internally accessible and usable to the patient and authorized personnel within a provider organization. A patient medical record implies a more comprehensive and longitudinal set of patient data accessible to a patient and authorized professionals in collaborating provider organizations. A patient health record includes these data and other information such as immunization records and changes in health status over longer periods of time.

Increased availability of patient information results in less paper, and continuously accessible EMRs will contribute to improved care delivery and patient safety. Historically, at least 20% of care delivery errors were associated with inaccessible or unavailable patient information when a provider and patient engage in a care delivery event. Instant access to relevant knowledge about a patient's history, medications, and problems is expected to substantially improve patient care delivery. Realization of such positive expectations will improve patient care, with quality, consistency, and continuity of patient care delivery at any time and any location with better precision, accuracy, and ultimately clinical outcomes.

Another important aspect of digitally transformed health care is enhanced clinical knowledge management, because traditional technology is not directly perceived as supporting clinical best practices.

Twenty-first century IT-driven healthcare computerization, automation, and simplification focuses on safety issues, because medication ordering and administration are especially error-prone, with frequent omission errors being more difficult to detect than commission mistakes. Thorough and deliberate transformation of professional practice and diligent change management must be tightly integrated with any process redesign and automation.

Senior leadership must first embrace and then develop and sustain deliberate care delivery process redesign. Organizational transformation and process digitalization encourage collaborative data, information, and knowledge sharing among and between provider and payer organizations, with senior management support.

Without leadership inspiration, comprehensive digital transformation benefits will not be achieved.

A digitally transformed provider organization is a reality with documented examples that demonstrate quantifiable operational benefits of this strategy.

Although perceived by some as daunting, most newly built facilities enjoy wholesale digitization as easier, with more efficiency and cost savings than established facilities. Changing processes to exploit IT is more difficult than when tasks are deliberately digitized from the onset. Representative conclusions from these experiences include the following:

- Investment must be made not only in technology but also in process organization and transformation, especially in clinical settings. Such transformation requires visionary, strong, and dedicated leadership.
- Although not always quantified, achieved benefits include significant quality improvement, increased operational efficiencies, cost savings, revenue generation, and charge capture.

- Significant, broad, and pervasive clinical process automation is estimated to be increasing by at least 20% every 5 years in large provider organizations.
- An accelerating number of provider organizations have or are investing in substantial new construction or renovation, including more than 60% investing in comprehensive digital transformation.
- As provider interoperability, integration, and interconnectedness accelerates, additional benefits of digital transformation are quantified, acknowledged, and embraced as achievable, and increasing demands will encourage reluctant providers.

Progressive growth comes with increased infrastructure, systems, and application capability and competitive advantage (much like banking experienced increased growth with adoption of automatic teller machines, or ATMs, which have been used by the general public during the last 30 years). Such growth is not without precedent.

Initially, banks invested heavily, installing ATMs in many places but without an integrated network. After these ATMs were connected through interoperable networks, user convenience and efficiency expanded worldwide. An identical opportunity exists within, among, and between healthcare providers and healthcare-related organizations of all types. The potential from healthcare ITs can be driven by a "killer application" (e.g., PACS and CPOE) with capabilities to connect, communicate, and share data, information, and knowledge.

Adoption of IT advances and associated organizational culture changes take time. As with experiences in other industries (e.g., online banking), it may take years until most providers and patients become comfortable and are proficient users. However, with persistence, sustainable funding and incentive-driven progress America's current care delivery processes and limited level of patient engagement will seem archaic as we achieve President Bush's challenge to use an EMR by 2014.

Ultimately, effectively deployed ITs and digitally transformed processes lower healthcare costs. In our current antiquated and bureaucratic healthcare system, all patients are at an unacceptable level of dying or are incurring serious harm as the result of a medical error. Because traditional American healthcare providers have been slow to embrace widespread comprehensive use of available IT, even the most diligent patients can be victims of unintended clerical oversight. Effective digital transformation with the required comprehensive process redesign and substantial information technologic deployment requires significant financial and resource investment over time. Patient lives and provider financial viability is at stake. This is not just theoretical optimism but rather a proven fact. A recent federal study conservatively demonstrated that an interoperable healthcare network will save our country at least $80 billion a year.

Even in early implementation stages of mandated HIPAA transactions, most community hospitals expected to save at least a million dollars annually from standardization and automation of only eight financial transactions, patient eligibility, claims, remittances, and so on. Such substantial cost savings are then applied to advancing and subsidizing other areas of healthcare delivery. These facts demonstrate intrinsic value of a more quality-driven, effective, digitally transformed healthcare delivery system.

Throughout history around the world, dramatic "cultural changes" in any aspect of business, government, or society began with a plan. Acceptance and adoption of IT and digitally driven healthcare transformation is no different. This plan for the digital transformation of health care has a goal and a defined vision of widespread use of EMRs by 2014. This vision was delivered clearly so that each of us, providers and patients alike, can see how it fits within our own personal reality. Effective, accessible, and affordable health care is very important to everyone. The complex maze of intersecting and unfortunately all too frequently unsafe and ineffective processes is not necessary. Digital transformation with effective IT deployment will result in healthcare delivery that is safer, easier, more effective and efficient with higher quality and at lower cost.

As was unfortunately demonstrated during the Gulf States floods in 2005, millions of patient paper medical records were lost, resulting in devastating healthcare delivery degradation. This proved once again that our current paper-based delivery system is irrational in today's technologically advanced world.

A digitally transformed healthcare delivery system would not permit such a loss to occur with so many unhealthy ramifications. With an EHR, this will not happen again. Similarly, study after study has demonstrated that medical errors are prevented with an EMR. In this age of pervasive computing capabilities and continually advancing digital technology, our current paper-based health system is literally killing thousands of patients each year.

Without contemplating additional emerging technologies in similar detail, following is an overview of key patient-centric technologies already "in the pipeline." When used progressively, pervasively, and with foresight, pioneering providers and provider organizations are enjoying, evaluating, and opportunistically exploring these technologies. Further development and widespread adoption may transform care delivery throughout individual organizations and among organization as shared services by competitors within their service area and beyond, some sooner rather than later.

Following are but a few examples:

- Use a cell phone on an individual, prevention-focused, knowledge-intense, and innovative way to monitor diabetes via embedded technology within the cell phone's extra battery space. This technology reads blood sugar levels and reports results to the patient's physician via a wireless connection. Based on detected results the cell phone can alert the patient when follow-up testing or medication is prudent.

- Use a global positioning system to track Alzheimer's patients with a wristband that wirelessly connects with a monitor at a nursing station so that each patient may be tracked while freely moving about.
- Enable remote monitoring to anticipate needed care of an elderly or sick patient by using internal motion sensor technology in conjunction with alarms in their homes.

As these examples demonstrate, there are virtually unlimited opportunities to improve the quality of life as technology continues to advance care and extend everyone's lifespan.

Unfortunately, key challenges include:

- Lack of national standards
- Concerns over privacy
- Lack of interoperable technologies throughout the country
- Voluntary NHIN participation, with some private sector elements reluctant to share information
- Lack of comprehensive nationwide NHIN funding that includes all components

Examples of these and many other benefits of "early adoption" automation abound throughout our healthcare industry.

There are representative examples of emerging technologies that are in use. Speech recognition applications only require a short learning curve for clinicians to efficiently use them, and they dramatically change a transcriptionist's role from one of data entry to a more efficient and effective role of editing computerized voice to text. Although technical capability has existed for decades, expansion to all clinicians from simple single departmental specialized utilization limited by unique vocabulary and system dictionary building has been rare. Staffing of transcriptionists has been reduced (expressed as full-time equivalents) by using speech-recognition software.

CPOE

Other robust studies have provided many examples of early benefits of CPOE, such as fewer prescribing errors. CPOE is a key component of any digital health strategy and plays a significant role in patient safety programs. CPOE improves patient safety by reducing order transcription errors and by improving legibility of orders.

Integration of CPOE with decision support technology further contributes to patient safety because alerts and reminders can intercept potential errors, such as dosing errors, medication conflicts, and allergies.

Clinicians can e-prescribe prescriptions and related orders by inputting them electronically and then transmitting to an appropriate fulfilling pharmacy. Clinical decision supports each clinician (e.g., drug interaction flags and allergy-related information). E-prescribing eliminates hard-to-read handwritten prescriptions as well as errors in dispensing (such as wrong drug or contraindicated drug) that sometimes result.

Electronic clinical note applications incorporate information on each patient's demographics, medical history, physician/nurse notes, and/or follow-up orders.

Electronic laboratory orders computerize ordering of desired testing by clinicians, and electronic results with technologist authorization enables rapid receipt and review of results by clinicians. Usually, this process incorporates clinical decision support, such as highlighting results out of the normal range.

Availability of images (such as CT or magnetic resonance images) to authorized clinicians any time, anywhere makes electronically stored images available to all medical teams beyond the radiology department.

Electronic guideline-based intervention reminders assist clinicians by proactively suggesting care that is likely required based on evidence-based knowledge and patient-specific data.

RFID

Radiofrequency identification (RFID) use in the healthcare setting lags behind airline, retail, and pharmaceutical industry adoption of RFID technology to replace traditional bar coding. Various healthcare industry trade groups acknowledge that pioneering use of tagged unit packages for medicines and patient identification has demonstrated significant promise for health care, as has been seen from implementations in other industries.

One of many RFID methods of identification, includes serial number storage that identifies an individual, object, or other information on a microchip attached to an antenna. The chip and the antenna together are called an RFID transponder or an RFID tag. This antenna enables the chip to transmit identification information to a reader. The reader converts radiowaves reflected back for further processing.

As of this writing, an increasing number of hospitals required hardware and software investments to use readers in trauma centers to track patients with RFID tags attached to their ankles. The U.S. Navy using RFID at its Pensacola Fleet Hospital in Iraq is another example.

Following are two examples of early benefits resulting from digital process transformation in airline and retail applications.

- An RFID technology standard has been adopted worldwide so all airlines in all countries can read each other's tags embedded with an RFID chip, using secured ultra-high frequency radio signals to transmit a bag's identifying number. The business case itself was very strong when driven by broad adoption of electronic ticketing. During pilot testing, this application consistently demonstrated more than 99% accuracy in tag recognition. This performance represents a significant improvement from 80% to 90% historical accuracy experienced with bar-coded tags read by optical scanners (enough to increase this process to Six Sigma "world class" quality).
- Wal-Mart, with the largest supply chain in the world, tested this technology, but as of this writing temporarily suspended global usage until all suppliers also embrace this dramatic innovation. This application uses these RFID microchips attached to each pallet and merchandise box that comes into Wal-Mart to replace bar codes. RFID enables Wal-Mart to track any pallet or box at any stage in its supply chain and to know exactly what product comes from which manufacturer and locate it by expiration date. Currently, each tag costs approximately $0.20. Until mass production significantly reduces this cost, Wal-Mart is planning for RFID use to large boxes and pallets, not individual items.

Surgical Implants

Surgically implanted devices not limited to pacemakers are being developed. As of this writing, a surgically implanted device is being reviewed by an FDA advisory panel as the first of many implantable sensors now being developed.

Two examples:

- A diagnostic hemodynamic monitor by Medtronic Inc. measures pressure and monitors body temperature and heart rate. Based on "alert parameters," this information is instantly and wirelessly transmitted via Internet to a physician to monitor or advise therapeutic intervention (i.e., life-threatening congestive heart failure).
- Numerous companies are developing comparable sensors that report periodically (i.e., weekly, once or twice daily) or report based on programmed alert parameters. These devices do not send alerts enabling a doctor to check the data on a regular basis. A number of companies are developing similar sensors that could have far-flung implications (e.g., implantable insulin pumps).

Recently, researchers demonstrated a prototype silicon-based chip that produces laser beams, enabling laser-focused photons (light) rather than wires and electrons to move data between chips. This breakthrough technology removes a formidable limitation in microchip design and computer system design. As a result, high-speed data communications can increase at a phenomenal rate, enabling increased processing capability, power, and speed with diminishing cost. This breakthrough portends comparable growth as forecast by Moore's Law, as has been repeatedly demonstrated with computer hardware for more than 50 years.

When commercialized before the end of this decade, thousands of data-carrying light beams on industry standard chips will revolutionize communications, information systems, and ultimately healthcare IT. Lasers are already used to transmit high volumes of computer data over longer distances (between offices, cities, and across oceans, using fiber-optic cables). In current microchips data moves at great speed over the inside wires but then slow to a snail's pace when they are sent chip-to-chip inside a computer.

Fiber-optic networks have been used for decades to transmit data globally within data centers, in neighborhoods, and among cities and countries. Some organizations (e.g., U.S. Naval Medical Command Headquarters in Washington, DC) have enjoyed much faster and more reliable communications to the desktop. These laser chips will make quantum leaps in communication to and from individual homes at virtually no cost. This is a very reasonable expectation because, as of this writing, there are literally millions of miles of "dark fiber" (phenomenal amounts of unused excess capacity) embedded in a global infrastructure since the beginning of this century.

Similarily, next generation search engines are being developed. As of this writing, entire contents of millions of books, are now available and searchable online via the Internet. This "democratization of data and information" has already had a profound impact on society. Just as Google's founders understood in the late 1990s, billions of web pages were accumulating in "searchable" databases. Upon realizing that existing search engines searching via keys could not keep pace, mathematical algorithms enabled proprietary rankings of web pages. Such web page links assumed that more individuals were linked to certain contents on each page. This breakthrough enabled ranking technologies with capabilities to search based on analysis of page content. Clinicians are demanding comparable analytic capabilities to be embedded in healthcare IT applications.

IT spending is growing faster in health care than in most other industries, as hospitals look to control escalating costs through efficiencies driven by IT and organization-wide digital transformation. Provider and business coalitions are now demanding less proprietary IT and more open architecture development. Applications are being designed based on federally mandated standards, such as HIPAA transactions, Health Level Seven, CCOW, and "low cost, no cost, open source" operating systems (e.g., Linux). When tied to reimbursement incentives, IT investments and digitally redesign will yield "bottom line" savings of more than 50% as compared with legacy IT system deployments.

SUMMARY

This chapter introduced and explained terminology, tools, techniques, and concepts associated with key disruptive technologies empowering providers to respond to government and societal demands for dramatically improved, higher quality, lower cost, and more patient-centric healthcare delivery processes.

Fundamental concepts and content focused on

- NHII
- Digital systems continuum
- Clinical technology opportunities and challenges
- A DHC requiring multifaceted technologies
- Paradigm shifts with innovative conceptual constructs

CHAPTER QUESTIONS

These questions reinforce student understanding, learning, and retention while stimulating class discussion:

1. Discuss current status of initiatives to achieve an EMR by 2014.
2. Identify benefits expected from organization-wide deployment PACS and CPOE.
3. How are emerging technologies and health care transformation related?
4. How will laser microchips improve health care?
5. How are airline and retail applications of RFID related to expected use in health care?
6. Which emerging technologies are likely to be in widespread use in other industries before 2014?
7. Which emerging technologies are likely to be in widespread use in healthcare industries before 2014?
8. Which two technologies demonstrate dramatic improvements in healthcare delivery?
9. Which technologies have already shown substantial process and care delivery transformation in pioneering provider organizations?
10. How is this chapter's content related to the content of other chapters in this book?

ADDITIONAL RESOURCES

These references are recommended for additional reading and more comprehensive content beyond the scope of this book.

Barry, R., Murcko, A., Brubaker, C. (2002). The Six Sigma Book for Healthcare. Chicago: Health Administration Press.

Bassard, M., Ritter, D. (1994). The Memory Jogger: A Pocket Guide of Tools for Continuous Improvement and Effective Planning. Salem, NH: Goal/QPC.

Coile, Jr., R. (2002). New Century Healthcare Strategies for Providers, Purchasers, and Plans. Chicago: Health Administration Press.

Coile, Jr., R. (2002). The Paperless Hospital: Healthcare in a Digital Age. Chicago: Health Administration Press.

Dale, N., Lewis, J. (2004). Computer Science Illuminated. Sudbury, MA: Jones and Bartlett.

Deming, W. E. (1986). Out of Crisis. Boston, MA: MIT Press.

Deming, E. Quality and Statistical Process Control. Cambridge, MA: MIT Center for Advanced Engineering Study.

Department of Health and Human Services. (2007). NHII Status. Retrieved June 29, 2007 from http://www.hhs.gov/go/healthit

Goldsmith, J. (2003). Digital Medicine Implications for Healthcare Leaders. Chicago: Health Administration Press.

Griffith, J., White, K. (2002). The Well-Managed Healthcare Organization. Chicago: Health Administration Press.

Harrell, C., Bateman, R., Gogg, T., Mott, J. (1996). System Improvement Using Simulation. Orem, UT: Promodel Corporation.

Herzlinger, R. (1997). Market-Driven Health Care: Who Wins, Who Loses in the Transformation of America's Largest Service Industry. Reading, MA: Perseus Books.

Ishikawa, K. (1985). Cause and Effect: The Japanese Way. Englewood Cliffs, NJ: Prentice-Hall.

Juran, J.M., Godrey, A.B. (1999). What Is Quality Control? New York: McGraw-Hill.

Larson, J. (2001). Management Engineering. Chicago: Healthcare Information and Management Systems Society.

Longest, Jr., B., Rakich, J., Darr, K. (2004). Managing Health Services Organizations and Systems. Baltimore, MD: Health Professions Press.

MacInnes, R. (2002). The Lean Enterprise Memory Jogger: Create Value and Eliminate Waste Throughout Your Company. Salem, NH: Goal/QPC.

Martin, P., Tate, K. (1997). Project Management Memory Jogger: A Pocket Guide for Project Teams. Salem, NH: Goal/QPC.

Nelson, R. (1999). Tele-health: Changing healthcare in the twenty-first century. Journal of Health Information Management, 13(4).

Newell, L. (2000). Beyond year 2000: Innovative solutions for the evolving healthcare information management environment. Journal of Health Information Management, 14(1).

Null, L., Lobur, J. (2006). The Essentials of Computer Organization and Architecture. Sudbury, MA: Jones and Bartlett.

Seidel, L., Gorsky, R., Lewis, J. (1995). Applied Quantitative Methods for Health Services Management. Baltimore, MD: Health Professions Press.

Seymour, D. (2006). Futurescan Healthcare Trends and Implications: 2006–2011. Chicago: Health Administration Press.

Tufte, E. (1990).Visual Explanations. Cheshire, CT: Graphics Press.

Tufte, E. (1997). Envisioning Information. Cheshire, CT: Graphics Press.

Tufte, E. (1997). The Visual Display of Information. Cheshire, CT: Graphics Press.

Veney, J., Kaluzny, A. (1998). Evaluation and Decision Making for Health Services. Chicago: Health Administration Press.

Wan, T. (1995). Analysis and Evaluation of Health Care Systems: An Integrated Approach to Managerial Decision Making. Baltimore, MD: Health Professions Press.

CHAPTER 16

Visionary Perspectives: Healthcare's Future . . . 2014 and Beyond

This chapter highlights near-term, expert-level healthcare industry forecasts of specific expectations of healthcare delivery digitalization. Key strategies and tactical approaches necessary for effective organizational transformation are summarized, emphasizing critical challenges and future opportunities for healthcare providers.

Strategies for healthcare's digital transformation demand a multi-disciplinary focus on comprehensive, pervasive delivery process redesign enabled by online, real-time, always-on, interoperable, interdependent, integrated, patient-centric IT systems and applications.

Transformational ITs digitize current technology and instruments on seamlessly integrated data networks to enable real-time clinician access into each patient's longitudinal EMR. Digitally advanced hospitals have demonstrated reduced lengths of stay, increased quality of care, and increased reimbursement. Computer hardware and software vendors and system integrators, all with reputations for effective design, project management, and implementation of complex systems in other service industries, joined with these hospitals to collaborate, develop, and support very early versions of "patient information systems."

El Camino Hospital's digital transformation experiences were detailed as representative healthcare information system characteristics and as rich functions and features effectively deployed for more than 50 years. At that time the Hospital provided emergency room care and diagnostic procedures for patients referred by staff physicians. This prototype system was a true hospital-wide system designed to store patient and financial data and to aggregate and communicate appropriate data and information, either automatically or upon request. Hospital objectives for this first-generation patient care information system included provision of more efficient healthcare delivery and improved patient care by facilitating and enhancing nursing and ancillary department activities. This successful "demonstration project" led to other large-scale data processing applications in medicine and health record systems, as computer growth accelerated in other industries. Hospitals began to justify additional system investment and then demonstrated continuing productivity gains and early evidence of increased process efficiency.

Technology is applied to every facet of clinical and business operations (e.g., integrating patients, personnel, process, technology, and cultural elements). IT is now defined more broadly as healthcare providers go beyond advanced clinical systems to include fundamental patient-centric integration and digital transformation of strategic processes associated with information and medical technologies.

Recent advances in information systems, networks, and telecommunication technologies enable global real-time collaboration and consultation among and between physicians and other members of the healthcare delivery team.

Information systems are a group of interoperable components, applications, and associated technologies operating computers and information systems and associated transformational applications, processes, and tasks. There is a multidisciplinary need for an integrated patient-centric digital transformation of healthcare delivery.

Chapter 2 introduced data collection topics, analytic techniques, and team dynamics tools.

Initial focus was on tools routinely used by management engineers, systems analysts, operations analysts, network engineers, process improvement teams, BPR task forces, and IT professionals of all disciplines who support the digital transformation of health care.

Flowcharts are used to document how a particular process or system functions and facilitates analyses to better understand and identify problems, delays, and potential process improvements. This aspect to process documentation is vital to ensure that all team members understand complete processes or workflows.

An "in-control" process can produce bad products. True process improvement results from balancing repeatability and consistency with the capability of meeting patient or customer requirements. Capability indices show a distribution of process results or outcomes in relation to patient or customer specifications. Meaningful trends or shifts can be identified while monitoring unusual events in a process that change average process performance.

Run charts enable teams to monitor performance to identify meaningful trends or shifts in average process performance and to track useful information.

Control charts are graphic representations of key characteristics of a process, showing plotted values of process performance with statistics derived from inherent process variation as control limits. Variation is the difference of output values of a process from the process mean.

Statistical process control uses of statistical techniques such as control charts to analyze process capability, output, or outcome. Appropriate action is required to achieve and sustain improved process capability.

Upon implementation of a proposed solution, control charts are then used to monitor process performance and sustain improved statistical process control over time.

"In control" does not imply that process outputs or outcomes meet system needs or patient expectations. Senior management must actively support opportunities to control and reduce variation in key organizational processes and systems. Was untrained staff involved in the process at any time? Could staff fatigue affect this process?

For mission critical processes, even processes under control may still be so broken that continuous process improvement or BPR projects will not produce acceptable outcomes. Process variation is dramatically reduced as this out of control process is brought under control.

Chapter 3 introduced IT and focused on key concepts such as IT capabilities, functions, features, memory, processing. Systems architecture strategically transform of IT-driven processes.

Related technology terminology about systems and applications of IT in current and future healthcare delivery processes is efficiently engineered to provide value and improve patient satisfaction with delivery organizations.

An operational understanding of computer systems of all types, patient demographics, and data analyses can rapidly produce information to support clinicians and computer-literate support staff with combined medical backgrounds and IT training. Unfortunately, significant technology investment over time has not been and is not now functionally integrated, nor does our current healthcare delivery support productive, patient-centered, effective, quality-driven, affordable healthcare delivery.

These common elements are required in all computer systems to perform data processing and transform data into useful information. Effective digital transformation of healthcare delivery processes depends on systems of all types. Data are collected, processed, and stored to meet perceived needs of a processes, functions, applications, or programs. Data are processed by computer systems controlled by programs directing this digital transformation into useful information for analysis and action.

Data are input to memory of a computer system via input devices and processed in a system's central processing unit. Upon completion of data processing, output as information may be used as produced or processed further through other computer programs or applications. Information results from data or facts collected and are processed in some manner.

Software is a set of programmed instructions directing system hardware components to complete data processing tasks. Systems software controls operation of a system, directing, commanding, scheduling, and confirming data processing functions performed. Applications software includes programs performing specific data processing functions for end-user functions.

Output may become input for further processing operations, resulting in a data processing cycle.

Hardware is any physical component used in a system to process data, such as a central processing unit, memory, keyboard, mouse, display, buses, printers, and displays. Hardware includes devices required for input, output, processing, and storage of data. Flash drives and optical storage technologies have dramatically increased data storage capabilities of virtually all computer systems.

A data processing cycle refers to each stage of data transformation into information. Processing refers to data manipulation that occurs in the computer's central processing unit to produce output (information). Processing may occur in different time frames. Off-line processing takes place at intervals so that information is not always current and not readily available in real time. Online systems are real-time systems in which processing takes place immediately so that upon input information is current.

Information system operations produce information by processing data include calculations, input, output, query, classifications, sorting, updating, summarizing, storage, and retrieval.

Online processing is real-time interactive or transaction data processing without any delay because processing occurs immediately upon the availability of input and output transactions. Processing of input transactions and processes usually occurs in transaction input sequence order. Online processing occurs through a direct connection between terminals and a computer system. Off-line processing systems do not provide direct communication with a computer's processing unit. Online systems are connected to a processing unit via batch processing and occur via an off-line application or system that stores data for processing at periodic intervals. Batch processing is a relatively inexpensive and efficient method for processing large data sets.

Data manipulation, aggregation, and organization reflect data transformation into meaningful information using basic data processing operations. Brief descriptions of these fundamental basic data processing operations follow. Regardless of input device used, data input must occur before other data processing operations can occur. Patient care information systems are designed so that authorized users specify and run these reports as needed with a "report writer."

Computers are defined and classified as various types of electronic devices capable of rapidly and reliably processing and transforming data into information. Information systems are functional applications or units working together to perform data processing task. These systems are classified by size (supercomputers as largest and mainframe computers are large computer systems capable of rapidly processing very large volumes of data). When processing has been performed and output is available, information is a product. Digital computers process bits and bytes.

Implied levels of state of the art IT capabilities were described as HEPIS. This comprehensive healthcare IT configuration is minimally necessary to provide effective, patient-centric, state of the art healthcare information management system functions and features. This level of system functions and features is required to support effective digital transformation of care delivery processes throughout a typical healthcare provider organization. HEPIS supports research and population analyses and facilitates patient access to data and sharing of information to improve data quality, consistency, and integrity in a securely networked environment throughout multiple provider entities within an integrated healthcare delivery system. Data in HEPIS are organized in a format supportive of timely, effective, and efficient care delivery in virtually any venue, regardless of patient or provider location or patient clinical information. These applications, modules, functions, and features transparently support patient-centric care delivery processes throughout HEPIS by using industry standard interfaces in an interoperable integrated network environment.

An "e-health" application supports a variety of customer-friendly patient-centric capabilities, including prescription refills, appointment scheduling, online forms completion, patient and provider access to health records, online health assessment tools, and high-quality real-time health information. HEPIS provides significant additional benefits beyond seamless automated support of care delivery in that it provides information to support demographic research and population analyses and facilitates patient access to data. Information sharing truly enables an IDS by improving data quality and security and minimizing mundane administrative costs.

Multidisciplinary applications of integrated patient-centric digital communication transformation in healthcare delivery are well-defined rules controlling how data are formatted and processed and then used in many different healthcare delivery networks. Hospitals with reportedly superior care delivery continue to improve to preserve their competitive edge. Average hospitals must improve care delivery quality to be recognized as an improving organization striving to become a superior provider of high-quality patient care.

Virtually all basic QM tools are used in process design, process redesign, process improvement, BPR, and Six Sigma initiatives. QM is a management philosophy that is process focused to commit organizational resources in a patient-centric, team-driven, collaborative environment. Patient-centric quality care must become a central systemic focus to use these tools and techniques to digitally transform processes, applications, and systems.

Deming's classic strategy is built on an organization-wide systemic understanding and reduction of process variation to improve quality to

- *Increase* quality and productivity while constantly decreasing costs by systematically and consistently improving systems, processes, and services to establish and maintain contemporary techniques and processes with training and supervision
- *Provide* process improvement tools and techniques that increase workforce productivity and develop pride of workmanship
- *Delegate* responsibility and authority to improve processes to those actually doing work by creating multidisciplinary cross-functional work teams responsible for design, development, and improvement of policies, procedures, processes, and systems
- *Commit* to measuring and monitoring patient care delivery quality by establishing process, results, and outcome measures and develop measures with patients and internal and external customers
- *Manage* processes by linking quality to existing strategic planning, management, and performance systems, striving for excellence with recognition, reward, and celebration
- *View* all care delivery as processes and make continuous improvements to better meet patient needs by benchmarking to innovate and achieve process improvement breakthroughs
- *Facilitate* continuous and breakthrough process improvement

Quality improvement is a process beginning with identification of chronic quality problems.

Nonconformance costs likely represent 25% to 30% of organization costs. Provider organizations can minimize these costs by focusing on process improvement, error-cause removal, employee training and retraining, management leadership, and organization-wide awareness of quality problems.

Benchmarking is a straightforward process used to develop new perspectives on care delivery processes and systems, patient needs, or requirements of other customers. Experts consider benchmarking as a structured process for gaining new perspectives on the needs of patients and work processes by identifying, measuring, and emulating best practices of service organizations both inside and outside the healthcare industry. The objective of benchmarking in healthcare provider organizations is to improve work processes by identifying, analyzing, and emulating best practices used inside and outside of healthcare organizations.

BPR is the fundamental rethinking and radical redesign of business processes as measures of performance, such as cost, quality, service, and speed. BPR teams analyze existing processes to learn and understand what is critical in each component that contributes to overall process performance. Preconceived notions are discarded and each process is viewed from a patient's perspective to fix rather than change a process. The focus is on processes, ignoring everything except process redesign.

The Department of Veterans Affairs is an excellent model of digital transformation in process. The VA has controlled costs while significantly improving quality. A recent congressionally mandated study concluded that VA patients received 15% more recommended care than patients served by non-VA providers. Specifically, the Rand Corporation reportedly found that VA patients received 67% of recommended care, whereas patients outside the VA system received only 51% of recommended services.

Subsequent chapters provided essential insight, information, and ideas necessary to effectively lead a digital transformation of care delivery processes to direct efficient and timely patient and medical information flow through technology-driven organizational performance. When this happens, care providers are more focused on effective patient care, not frustrated by poor patient and process flow that inevitably leads to sub par clinical outcomes. Visible, committed, constant communication of the urgent need for operational change is necessary to achieve the organization's mission and vision of digital transformation. Realization of these goals is demonstrated by improved patient and staff experience resulting from improved patient and process flow by effective clinicians and other participants.

Existing systems, processes, procedures, tasks, or jobs in healthcare organizations were frequently developed by other industries. Process redesign team members should encourage constructive critical review and candid feedback to ensure that all system and process stakeholders, owners, and users understand and accept recommended process and technology changes with proposed solutions. Five classic work simplification techniques—work distribution, flow process, time flow analysis, horizontal flow process analysis, and job sequencing—were explained with examples of metrics for parameters such as patient volume, service time, and staffing levels. Cost-effective improvement is necessary in virtually every processing component of any delivery process to reduce patient waiting and server idle time. Productivity is improved while simultaneously reducing service delivery cost.

Examples of high priority mission critical functions were identified as patients waiting for service, laboratory specimens waiting for processing, analysis and result reporting, patient accounts waiting for third-party reimbursement, and patient dunning cycles. Idle servers are not productive components of any healthcare delivery system. As resources are added to a service process (adding an additional clinician or support staff member), service speed or processing rate can increase the number of patients simultaneously evaluated and treated in this process.

If surgery demand is greater than three operating rooms supporting surgery on three patients at one time, some patients must wait. Legacy healthcare delivery processes or systems were designed with an average productivity of 80%, and a "surge capacity" of potentially 90%. Clinical acceptability or unacceptability of delay in any process in any care delivery system providing demanded service varies based on clinical and medical considerations. Effective application of IT can digitally transform these aspects of care delivery dramatically.

These improvements fundamentally alter patient perspectives and significantly increase patient satisfaction. Most healthcare processes are complex and therefore reflect multiple services provided by multiple servers:

• Patient acceptance of delay, affecting patient participation in this or future service
• Average number of patients in process
• Average time a patient spends in process, including both waiting and service time
• Average number of patients in queue waiting for service

In a single-channel single-server system an idle system means an idle server (no patients experiencing any wait for service); whereas a busy system means that a patient must wait for service. Probability of a specific number of patients in a service process is defined by the average number of patients in process, average time each patient spends waiting and served in process, average time each patient is in queue, percentage of time, or probability that an arriving patient must wait for service. Incorporated with additional information on service costs and patient waiting line limitations (space), systems analysts, operations analysts, management engineers, and operations managers use process improvement tools to analyze, design, and iteratively redesign waiting lines. Analytical systems support Poisson probability distribution analyses of patient arrivals and throughput processing. Bottlenecks in processes must be identified and options evaluated through analysis of arrival times, process length, service departure times, etc.

Direct care or service costs must appropriately address key aspects of "hands-on" patient care; diagnostic, therapeutic, or nursing costs necessary to incorporate all resource requirements; and infrastructure and related expenses necessary for all aspects of well-managed patient care delivery. As provider organization's reorganize and refine processes and staffing patterns, effective use of a well-designed productivity management system facilitates appropriate resource allocation. Without credible functioning productivity management systems, department managers and senior executives will find this process very difficult, if not impossible.

Increasing healthcare costs are continuing to challenge providers to streamline operations by continuous process improvement, BPR, and so on, as leaner budgets are inevitable. Information produced using these productivity metrics provide data used to identify and develop future budgets and ongoing future process improvement opportunities. Obviously, staffing analyses are a direct result of applying productivity information to specific processes or departments.

Interest in process simulation and predictive modeling has increased substantially as contemporary techniques have been recognized as vital tools to support digital transformation of healthcare processes. Most of this renewed interest has been associated with increasing interest by healthcare organizations embracing QM, continuous process improvement, BPR, and Six Sigma and Lean enterprise initiatives.

For example, facilities of a hospital, such as staff, physicians and administrative personnel, diagnostic instruments, and information systems, are examples of relatively self-contained healthcare system components at one level and parts of a larger healthcare system at another level, possibly overall health care delivery in a city or county. Simulation and predictive modeling of healthcare delivery process or system changes typically use patients arriving for urgent unscheduled emergent care. Process modeling and simulation can educate team members, senior management, and "process owners" on current system operations and how a system might respond to alternative courses of action.

Six Sigma study focuses on DMAIC objectives that measurably improve key patient services and associated key processes. Digitally transformed patient care delivery systems, processes, and related operational applications demonstrate ongoing, consistent, and fundamentally improved performance. Six Sigma initiative sponsors must reinforce breakthrough performance with tangible rewards and recognition. Integrating Six Sigma tools and techniques into performance improvement must address cultural belief systems with disciplined project management expertise because current healthcare processes only operate at Six Sigma levels 2 through 3. Edward Deming's rationale for statistical process control emphasized increased control over process variation. Significant error reduction is achieved, quality of care delivery is improved, and cost savings result.

Lean principles reduce the waste that is pervasive in America's healthcare system. The IHI believes that adoption of Lean management strategies, although challenging, will likely enable healthcare organizations to improve processes and outcomes, reduce cost, and increase patient, provider, and staff satisfaction. "Pull" rather than "push" transformation system design is encouraged to improve care delivery pace and associated processes. Effective systematic digital transformation improves process efficiency and effectiveness by eliminating waste, reducing delays and costs, and improving quality.

Lean strategy incorporates the concept of "pull versus push" systems and processes. This unique approach has advantages to be considered as new systems and processes are designed, developed, and implemented or as legacy systems are improved or redesigned through Six Sigma, QM, or BPR initiatives. Pull systems deliver patient care services or related products promptly when and as requested by "downstream" processes or requirements. Pull systems reflect a streamlined flow of patient care services with more efficient delivery than push processes. Pull systems and component processes are used extensively in Lean enterprise organizations. Alternatively, push systems incorporate less efficient patient care delivery processes. Improvement teams can determine potential opportunities in care delivery processes and related system components to achieve expected performance goals as demonstrated by unacceptable "takt" times.

Takt time represents an expected rate at which healthcare provider systems and processes must operate to meet demand requirements. Historically, multidisciplinary initiatives that engaged information systems designers, operations analysts, and management engineers have not been chartered to produce integrated "future state" solutions that add significant value to IT investments, networks communications, and diagnostic and therapeutic technologies to address "current state" shortcomings of our healthcare delivery systems. By using a "who, what, where, when and how" approach red flag high opportunity functions are identified:

- Patient or personnel movement, including transport
- Movement of material, information, or technology
- Patient care or delivery process decision-making

Patients have not and are not experiencing patient-centric integrated information systems, communications technologies, and effectively transformed processes as are to be expected from seamless delivery systems. As integrated multidisciplinary strategies and tactics are applied through effective digital transformation, results from successful transformations include cost reductions of 25% to 55%, quality improvements or defect reductions of 50% to 90%, and lead time reductions of 50% to 90%.

Early-adopter organizations have demonstrated that effective digital transformation of patient care delivery produces quantum advances in diagnostic and therapeutic care with comprehensively integrated systems, applications, and finely-tuned supportive processes.

Informatics embodies an ever-expanding set of dedicated and specialized applications of IT to patient care delivery processes and research, including computer capabilities and staff throughout healthcare provider and research organizations.

Current initiatives focus on these key concepts:

- E-health applications
- HDSS
- DW
- DM

These applications are enabling providers to diagnose and treat patients and deliver ongoing care with significantly improved quality, efficiency, effectiveness, and safety. Clinicians are more effectively monitoring patient-centric care delivery and developing innovative new therapies throughout and beyond traditional provider networks. Health informatics and telemedicine emphasizes clinical and biomedical applications of e-health technologies. During the last decade interest expanded in a variety of settings, such as e-medicine, administrative, clinical, e-commerce, and financial applications of e-health and other e-clinical decision support and expert systems. Use of e-nursing support systems and other e-health applications such as e-home care systems, intelligent medical information systems, and HDSS have increased and accelerated.

In the context of this revolutionary diffusion of these IT-driven tools, e-health is a true paradigm shift from a physician- and clinician-centered delivery system to a consumer-driven patient-centric system (e-health systems that focus on patients rather than on caregivers).

Through informatics applications patients now have ready access to creditable world-class information sources:

- VPRs and networked electronic imaging can document communication, storage, and retrieval management capabilities.
- GIS are powerful tools for collecting, recording, storing, manipulating, and displaying spatial data sets.
- HDSS bundles analytic modeling, network communications, and decision technology to support group decision-making processes (strategic thinking, problem formulation, and generation of goal-seeking solutions).

From a clinician's perspective, rapid developments are driven from accelerated innovations in HDSS, clinical decision support systems, and expert decision support systems. From an administrator's perspective, rapid developments are driven from accelerated innovations like EIS, DW, and DM.

Published comparative information about the most efficient and effective healthcare providers to individual consumers and group purchasers of health services, business coalitions and patients are increasing transparent benchmarks for healthcare cost and quality. Accelerating availability of this information in a public forum is one more incentive for leaders in provider organizations to sponsor and fully support aggressive digital transformation initiatives. Additional incentives, opportunities, and threats abound.

Successful e-health system planning also requires management of the entire technologic infrastructure and information processing capacity of virtual business systems. Senior leadership must embrace these visionary concepts to ensure that information resources and e-technology are best adapted to meet patient and care provider needs. E-health system planning, implementation, and evaluation include incorporation of e-health transactional activities into virtual e-health systems, training and education of users migrating from legacy systems to e-health systems.

E-health impacts individual clinicians, system users, and patients via virtual alliances, workgroups, management, interactions, networking capabilities, and collaborative decision-making. For example, a VPR that is accessible by multiple care providers integrates patient history of diagnoses, treatments, and other therapeutic information from different providers regarding each patient. These impacts of e-health systems will eventually extend to the entire healthcare delivery system at both a community and societal level.

As the pace and intensity of these "disruptive technologies" accelerate, hospitals, other healthcare provider organizations, and individual healthcare workers are migrating toward e-health delivery models requiring government, public, and provider support and collaboration.

Evolving examples include:

- NHII
- Digital systems continuum
- Clinical technology opportunities and challenges
- DHC

A digital hospital is a point of a continuum as healthcare delivery organizations incrementally automate their core processes. Advanced clinical information systems improve patient safety and quality of care because clinicians are less distracted and can spend their time with patients rather than searching for radiology images, reports, or laboratory results. Providers must focus management attention to deep process redesign, as with any business process engineering initiative, to ensure expected benefits from any significant IT project to be realized.

More health care occurs in communities than in hospitals. IT management is a strategic benefit. With diligent and disciplined digital transformation, an effective foundation is built upon which IT investments will rapidly demonstrate focus and care delivery quality, efficiency, and effectiveness. Adoption of IT advances and associated organizational culture changes take time. Ultimately, effectively deployed ITs and digitally transformed processes lower healthcare costs. Sustained healthcare delivery provider viability will be led by digitally transformed information-enabled organizations delivering patient-centric care with advanced imaging modalities and interventional devices.

These progressive collaborative provider organizations will enjoy better capabilities to deliver more effective, higher quality, lower cost care. They will continue to thrive as IT advances demonstrate ongoing clinical benefits and increased patient satisfaction accrues from the digital transformation of care delivery driven by IT investment.

FAST FORWARD TO 2014

By achieving the goals established by President G. W. Bush's challenge to have fully implemented EMRs, a foundation for a very bright future is on the horizon. As an industry, health care will have moved beyond the "nuts and bolts" phase detailed in earlier chapters to digitally transform all aspects of care delivery. The following list presents but a few realistic expectations from recognized healthcare futurists. Each of these "predictions" is predicated on a digitized personal health record that is fully accessible from anywhere any time by a patient and any authorized clinician. Although most of these expectations require significant technologic advancements in many other fields, healthcare IT professionals are challenged to plan, execute, and evaluate the care delivery aspects associated with these longer term goals.

Digitized health care is in a "discovery phase" and considered by many visionaries as quite primitive. Physicians, clinicians, and other healthcare professionals expect to enjoy future iterations of innovations paralleling digital transformation experiences in other industries. Emerging technologies, beyond those highlighted in Chapter 15, are necessary precursors of that yet to come. These technologies will evolve at the nexus of healthcare delivery, ITs, informatics, nanotechnology, and cognitive science.

This list is presented as a "wish list" without benefit of detailed definition or specification. This limited level of clarity, accuracy, or precision is commonly associated with predictions of events that have not yet occurred, much like simulation and predictive modeling explained in Chapter 11:

- Personalized medicine includes pharmacogenomics derived from DNA and data mined with decision support tools like those described in Chapters 11 through 14. Engineered DNA is already enabling personalized medicine as scientists explore new options in life and human performance.
- Health enhancement and longevity is enabling a longer life with more vitality. Realistic expectations are that within the next decade a centurion will be the rule rather than the exception. While recognizing that Socrates was very insightful but dead before the age of 30, this generation is living longer than any humans in history.
- Health informatics is already enhancing healthcare information delivery. Ultimately these applications are key tools to controlling costs and increasing healthcare delivery efficiency.

- Infinite networks are increasingly commonplace, with phenomenally powerful computers that routinely operate 24 hours, 7 days a week to create next generation treatments.
- Stem cell and therapeutic cloning are not yet beyond a breakthrough phase. Who knows what our future will hold.

As one might expect, "decision-making with uncertainty" is nothing when compared to forecasting health status. Comprehensive "future health" incorporates predicting future disease states, or restoring cognition, bones, muscles, and organs to sustain productivity through a longer healthier life. But then, that's another book not yet written.

Bibliography

Barry, R., Murcko, A., Brubaker, C. (2002). The Six Sigma Book for Healthcare. Chicago: Health Administration Press.

Bassard, M., Ritter, D. (1994). The Memory Jogger: A Pocket Guide of Tools for Continuous Improvement and Effective Planning. Salem, NH: Goal/QPC.

Caldwell, C. (1998). The Handbook for Managing Change in Healthcare. Milwaukee, WI: Quality Press.

Coile, Jr., R. (2002). New Century Healthcare Strategies for Providers, Purchasers, and Plans. Chicago: Health Administration Press.

Coile, Jr., R. (2002). The Paperless Hospital: Healthcare in a Digital Age. Chicago: Health Administration Press.

Crosby, P. (1979). Quality Is Free. New York: McGraw-Hill.

Dale, N., Lewis, J. (2004). Computer Science Illuminated. Sudbury, MA: Jones and Bartlett.

Deming, W. E. (1986). Out of Crisis. Boston, MA: MIT Press.

Department of Health & Human Services. (2007). NHII status. Retrieved June 29, 2007 from http://www.hhs.gov/go/healthit/

Gogg, T., Mott, J. (1996). System Improvement Using Simulation. Orem, UT: Promodel Corporation.

Goldsmith, J. (2003). Digital Medicine: Implications for Healthcare Leaders. Chicago: Health Administration Press.

Griffith, J., White, K. (2002). The Well-Managed Healthcare Organization. Chicago: Health Administration Press.

Hammer, M., Champy, J. (2001). Reengineering the Corporation. New York: HarperCollins Publisher.

Harrell, C., Bateman, R., Gogg, T., Mott, J. (1996). System Improvement Using Simulation. Orem, UT: Promodel Corporation.

Herzlinger, R. (1997). Market-Driven Health Care: Who Wins, Who Loses in the Transformation of America's Largest Service Industry. Reading, MA: Perseus Books.

Ishikawa, K. (1985). Cause and Effect: The Japanese Way. Englewood Cliffs, NJ: Prentice-Hall.

Juran, J.M., Godrey, A.B. (1999). What Is Quality Control? New York: McGraw-Hill.

Labovitz, G. (1997). The Power of Alignment. Billerica, MA: Organizational Dynamics.

Larson, J. (2001). Management Engineering. Chicago: Healthcare Information and Management Systems Society.

Longest, Jr., B., Rakich, J., Darr, K. (2004). Managing Health Services Organizations and Systems. Baltimore, MD: Health Professions Press.

MacInnes, R. (2002). The Lean Enterprise Memory Jogger: Create Value and Eliminate Waste Throughout Your Company. Salem, NH: Goal/QPC.

Martin, P., Tate, K. (1997). Project Management Memory Jogger: A Pocket Guide for Project Teams. Salem, NH: Goal/QPC.

Nelson, R. (1999). Tele-health: Changing healthcare in the twenty-first century. Journal of Health Information Management, 13(4), 3–120.

Newell, L. (2000). Beyond year 2000: Innovative solutions for the evolving healthcare information management environment. Journal of Health Information Management, 3(4), 71–77.

Null, L., Lobur, J. (2006). The Essentials of Computer Organization and Architecture. Sudbury, MA: Jones and Bartlett.

Seidel, L., Gorsky, R., Lewis, J. (1995). Applied Quantitative Methods for Health Services Management. Baltimore, MD: Health Professions Press.

Seymour, D. (2006). Futurescan Healthcare Trends and Implications: 2006–2011. Chicago: Health Administration Press.

Tufte, E. (1990). Visual Explanations. Cheshire, CT: Graphics Press.

Tufte, E. (1997). Envisioning Information. Cheshire, CT: Graphics Press.

Tufte, E. (1997). The Visual Display of Information. Cheshire, CT: Graphics Press.

Veney, J., Kaluzny, A. (1998). Evaluation and Decision Making for Health Services. Chicago: Health Administration Press.

Wan, T. (1995). Analysis and Evaluation of Health Care Systems: An Integrated Approach to Managerial Decision Making. Baltimore, MD: Health Professions Press.

Index